Guiding Principles of Natural Horse Care

Powerful Concepts for a Healthy Horse

Stephanie Krahl

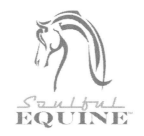

Soulful Creatures™ LLC

Published by Soulful Creatures™ LLC, dba Soulful Equine™

Web: www.soulfulequine.com - *Helping Your Horse Thrive™*

First edition: September 2011

ISBN: 978-0615617503

Horse head image on cover by Laurie Justus Pace.

Photos in book by Lynn McKay.

Trademarks and Service Marks

To those who choose to make changes to their horse care practices
so their horses will thrive and live a long, quality life.

CONTENTS

LEGAL INFORMATION

DISCLAIMER OF LIABILITY

The authors and publisher shall have neither liability nor responsibility to any person(s) or entities with respect to any loss or damage, caused or alleged to be caused directly or indirectly as a result of the information contained in this book, or appearing on the Soulful Equine website. While this book is as accurate as the authors can make it, there may be unintentional errors, omissions, and inaccuracies.

TERMS AND CONDITIONS

This book is for informational and educational purposes only. The information presented and contained within this book is based on the training and experience of the author. Its content is not intended to be used as a substitute for professional medical advice, diagnosis or treatment. **Always** consult your veterinarian for any medical concerns, questions or advice you may have regarding your animal. Reliance on any information provided by Soulful Equine is solely at your own risk.

PART I: CORE VALUES

No matter what decisions we make in our lives, those decisions will usually reflect our core values. Sometimes it's difficult to overcome our inner struggle to honor our values, especially when we are weighed down by external influences. It's time to overcome those struggles and make decisions that resonate with you and that are in your horse's best interest. This section will help you get started.

INSTABILITY AND FOUNDATIONAL STRUCTURE

"Great spirits have always encountered violent opposition from mediocre minds." ~ Albert Einstein

The intent of this book is to create a shift in your thinking that will empower you to become more confident when it comes to making difficult decisions that relate to your horse's health and well-being. You'll benefit from this shift in thinking if you're ready to make changes in your approach to horse guardianship. Alternatively, if you already keep your horse naturally but you'd like to optimize or look for any holes in your program, this will help.

Finally, if you're stuck in any way when it comes to keeping your horse naturally, this book is for you. You never know when you'll find a golden nugget of information that will help connect the dots or provide validation. Sometimes the comfort of validation is enough to empower us and build confidence in our abilities.

As you set out on this journey that goes against conventional beliefs, you'll encounter people who will come into your life and help you at just the right moment. On the other hand, you'll also encounter those who will try to prevent you from making necessary changes you feel are best for you and your horse. Their agenda is usually not in your best interest and, for that matter, is not in your horse's best interest either.

What it boils down to is that the decisions you make must resonate with you and line up with your core values.

THE CORE PRINCIPLE THAT SETS US UP FOR SUCCESS

Soulful Equine™ stands for prevention, quality of life and longevity with a mission of *Helping Your Horse Thrive*™. Our optimal model is the wild horse; however, it's impossible for a domesticated horse to ever reach such a level of soundness and health as that of a wild horse.

You may ask, "If it's impossible, then why should we learn about this model?" Although it seems to be impossible, that shouldn't keep us from getting as close as we can to an environment that mimics that of wild horses. Using that as our model, puts Mother Nature back in the driver's seat. It introduces guidelines to provide optimal health for our horses.

> *"The core principle that sets your horse up for optimal health is the concept of staying as close to nature's intent for the horse as possible, which means treat your horse as a horse, not how humans think a horse should be treated."*
> ~ Stephanie Krahl

Using that core principle as your basic foundation and belief system is essential. A great foundation is important to anything worth doing. Without it, what we've worked so hard for can easily collapse.

For example, if a building is constructed quickly and without a good foundation, it may develop problems over time. Eventually you may see cracks in the walls and leaks around the windows. The house shifts so much that it soon becomes unstable and finally must be condemned because it's no longer safe.

When it comes to horses, I believe in a solid foundation in all aspects of horse care. That includes, but is not limited to, horsemanship, nutrition, hoof care as well as the **mental, emotional and spiritual well-being** of the horse.

Without an understanding of foundational structure when it comes to your horse, she can't thrive and eventually she will end up like the house I described above. Her life with you may be cut short prematurely simply because you chose not to seek more knowledge.

However, if you're reading this book, you're not one of those people. Instead, you're one of the few who seek continuing education, so give yourself a pat on the back.

I DON'T WANT TO WASTE YOUR TIME

Before we continue, I want to make sure your time is not wasted. In order for me to make this book useful to you, I'm going to make some general assumptions based on the following fundamental principles:

1) You're open to new ideas that may be contrary to your current horse care philosophy and beliefs.
2) You understand that in order to succeed at anything you must first grasp and implement key fundamental concepts before moving on to advanced approaches.
3) You're open to continuous learning and self-improvement.
4) You genuinely care about your horse's quality of life and longevity.

Most people who implement a successful program that encourages a naturally healthy horse understand and utilize these principles. I'm going to go into each one in more detail.

1) You're open to new ideas that may be the opposite of your current beliefs about horse care.

One of the most difficult things for people is *change*. It's also difficult to find out one day that what you *thought* was right was really all wrong. The conflict occurs partly because of ego and external pressures and partly from feelings of inadequacy. It's human nature and a step in the learning process; however, it doesn't make it easier when change is involved.

It's important you understand up front that most of what you may learn will be the complete opposite of what you were either told or what is being taught by experts. It's critical that you remain open to new ways of approaching your horse care practices.

This doesn't mean you should believe new ideas without question, instead, carefully evaluate those ideas before closing your mind to them. What matters is that those ideas resonate with you once you consider them. Take from the information what applies to your situation and leave the rest.

2) You understand that in order to succeed at anything you must first grasp and implement key fundamental concepts *before* moving on to advanced approaches.

We've all had that feeling of wanting something *now*. The thing we want may look cool, slick or ideal, but in that moment of desire we're not thinking about what it takes to get there. Have you ever heard the saying, "The fancy stuff comes from having solid fundamentals?" In Neuro-linguistic programming (NLP) the principle is, "Repetition of the basics leads to mastery." Both of these statements apply to any endeavor in life that we pursue.

Not grasping core fundamental concepts can set us up for failure or, at best, accepting the status quo by being mediocre. This book is called *The Guiding Principles* for a reason. It provides a core foundation to build on. If you want all the advanced concepts and details now then this book is not for you.

3) You're open to continuous learning and self-improvement.

This particular statement usually weeds out a lot of people. The majority of people don't like change nor do they prefer to seek more knowledge. Keeping the status quo is the norm. By default, learning new concepts and working on yourself will invoke change in your life. Awareness is the first step.

If you're not willing to look in the mirror and acknowledge some truths, then your circumstances won't change. Therefore, your horse's situation will not change. If you're happy where you are then there's no reason to continue learning more... right? But you're here so something is motivating you to listen (maybe it's your horse).

4) You genuinely care about your horse's quality of life *and* longevity.

In this day and age it's all about the next blue ribbon or big futurity; it's not about the horse. The horse is secondary. If it doesn't work out with this horse, just sell her or dispose of her. That's usually the mentality.

I'm not just talking about older horses. I'm also considering the young horses that are tossed aside because they "didn't make it." It means either that they didn't win or, after going through training, it was agreed that they didn't have the physical or mental ability to compete successfully.

In reality, those horses were most likely misunderstood and the approach to their training was unfair and possibly even abusive. As long as they're treated as disposable objects for winning ribbons and money, horses will continue to be bred at alarming rates and treated inhumanely as merely a means to an end. This contributes to the over population of America's horses.

Although your horse must be "healthy" to compete, have you first considered whether or not her quality of life is optimal? Are her **body, mind** *and* **spirit** able to be sustained for the long haul? How long will your horse last without major issues as she grows older? That's the big question. If you don't care about both quality of life and longevity, then taking the natural horse care route may not be best for you, even though it *is* what's best for your horse.

Do any of these principles sound elementary? You may be surprised that their application is somewhat rare. When it comes to horses, many times fear, frustration and not knowing who to believe can create confusion. You may freeze and not move forward at all. It's just too much for most people.

Most people say they want to understand by starting with the fundamentals, but they don't practice it. They usually end up understanding "just enough" to get by and then move on to the next thing. That's like putting the roof on a house so you don't get rained on while you're pouring the slab for the foundation.

> *Almost any time problems arise, it's an indication that a fundamental concept was skipped in your approach to horse care.*

Grasping, understanding and applying the fundamentals in most anything will promote optimization. What does that mean? It means that once you master the basics, advancement will come much easier.

Do you think someone who has a black belt in karate started with a black belt? No, she learned the core fundamentals first, which sent her on her way to mastery. Of course, it's up to her to decide whether or not she wants to *seek* mastery. The same holds true for you.

It all depends on what you want in life and what kind of life you want for your horse. If you want to accept mediocrity, Soulful Equine is not for you. If you want to move forward, resolve reoccurring doubts and cause change in the world, then stick around and we would love to go down that road with you.

It won't offend me if you've found that this book is not for you. I would rather save you time since we're not a good match. If, however, what I've covered so far resonates with you, then I would like to invite you to join me on a journey to helping your horse thrive.

I do need to warn you, the guiding principles presented in this book have changed lives.

Many times it means drastic change for you and your horse. I have to say, I'm one of those people.

In the coming chapters, I'll share my story with you. But first, I'll begin by diving into the word "expert." I'll be the first to say I don't claim to have all the answers - that's what the experts are for, right? Don't they have all the answers?

THINK OF THE WORD "EXPERT" DIFFERENTLY

Seeking knowledge and learning more about how to properly care for your horse can be intimidating, especially when it's difficult to know who or what to believe.

There are no experts, only differing schools of thought, and people with a variety of experiences and levels of knowledge.

I believe the word "expert" is a meaningless term. Sometimes people are awarded that label merely because they possess credentials, and when these types of people get into positions of power, that label can be misused and abused.

Not everyone who is an authority in their field has credentials. The future of education lies in the hands of those who enjoy sharing their vast knowledge, years of experience and, most importantly, their ability to solve problems.

It's my intent to help you think of the word "expert" differently, at least in the sense of how it relates to the horse industry. I think we get so caught up in that word that it becomes problematic.

It boils down to whether or not you're able to help people solve a problem. I would much rather be known as someone who can help people solve problems instead of being called "an expert" in a certain subject.

The irony is that over time when you start to help people solve problems, you get a reputation of being an authority. The key point is, are you serving people with the greatest standard of care and providing value? Again, the question you have to ask before you think of someone as an expert is "are they able to help you solve problems?" I can think of many people who are considered experts who only *think* they're solving problems when, in reality, they're causing more problems.

> **In the truest sense of the term, "expert" means you've developed a competence and depth of knowledge in a specialized area.[1]**

Selecting an individual to assist you with your horse care needs should not be based *solely* on credentials. Nor should their having credentials be an eliminating factor in your choice. It's critical that you learn to balance the two and learn how to carefully choose who may best be able to help you.

It's important to note that, generally, the credentialed individual relies on science. Science *is* powerful. It's helped solve many problems in our modern world. The true power, however, is Mother Nature, and we humans would be best served if we used science to understand Her, rather than using it to manipulate Her.

Balancing the two is an *intuitive art* of which few are capable. Often the credentialed individual proceeds as though science is king, when in fact Mother Nature reigns.

---

1   Dictionary.com - paraphrased.
    <http://dictionary.reference.com/browse/expert> Accessed 2011.

"Nature has a built-in wisdom in every single detail of her creation, including us. We belong to the wisdom of nature; nature does not belong to us."[2] ~ *Caroline Myss*

We all have some kind of special skill or knowledge in some area. *We are all experts in our own lives.* We each experience events and feelings differently; no two experiences are identical. These differing experiences are what cause many controversial opinions in the horse industry. No one situation, horse, experience or solution is the same. This can make it difficult to know who to believe.

The simple answer is... your horse.

Through your horse, you will find answers to many of your questions. Your horse can be an excellent teacher if you're willing to listen and learn. Sometimes, while learning something new, you may experience a certain level of fear. Change alone can cause fear to arise, but fear is your friend. It not only protects you, but it can cause you to grow as an individual. In an upcoming chapter, I will touch on the subject of fear and how it relates to your horse's care.

THE BOOK MAP

Throughout this book, I'll share with you many of my experiences about horse care. The range of information will vary, but I will touch on key foundational concepts that are important to understand. Again, the goal is a good foundation that includes prevention focused on quality of life and longevity. Without that goal, circumstances will eventually produce an unfavorable outcome.

Something I've noticed in others who become empowered with knowledge is that the more they learn the more they want to share. Naturally, knowledge leads to confidence and empowerment. A valuable lesson I've learned over the years is the power in setting good examples. This approach will keep you from forcing your new-found knowledge, beliefs and ideas on to someone else. It's a powerful

---

2   Caroline Myss, "The Profound Order of Nature." 25 May 2011
    <http://www.myss.com/news/archive/2011/052511.asp>.

approach especially when it comes to horses. Setting good examples is stronger than any traditional teaching method. So, hold back on those reins a little and do your best to contain yourself when you obtain knowledge you feel can change people's or horses' lives. I will dive deeper into this concept in the coming chapters.

WHAT TO FOCUS ON

There are no quick fixes when it comes to having a naturally healthy horse. If you ever feel overwhelmed when learning new information, such as what is presented in this book, give yourself permission to focus on only what applies best to your horse and situation.

GENERAL BOOK OVERVIEW

This book is made up of a collection of key natural horse care concepts published on the Soulful Equine website over the years. It includes modifications to those articles along with additional materials that expand on certain subjects such as nutrition, hoof care and other overall natural horse care concepts mixed with a little personal development.

If you're not sure what natural horse care is all about, this book will point you in the right direction to understanding horses from their point of view and how you can honor their natural state. Keep in mind that there's nothing "natural" about keeping horses in domestication.

Rather, think of natural horse care as the horse care concepts you implement in order to maintain a healthy horse in mind, body and spirit. This will in-turn result in quality of life and longevity.

So, sit back and enjoy the journey. I hope you'll obtain additional knowledge from the information I share with you throughout this book.

WHAT THIS BOOK DOES NOT COVER

This book doesn't dive into the details of every aspect of natural horse care. Natural horse care is a huge subject. An introduction to important key concepts and foundational information is provided, no more, no less.

PART II: PREVENTION VERSUS DISEASE

The word "prevention" is not in most people's vocabulary especially when it comes to horses. Those who have little or no respect for Mother Nature and other living creatures don't usually combine these two words, prevention and horses. Instead, it's usually about the next big futurity or blue ribbon. The horse is secondary.

For most people, winning is more important than having core values. Usually, core values are nowhere in the equation.

What if we found an almost perfect balance between the two so we could have both? The following chapters will help you understand some core principles that will get you closer to that ideal.

THE FEAR OF NOT CONFORMING

*"When you resist your fears, they become stronger.
Acknowledge their presence and they will have
less hold on you."* ~ Denise Linn

WHAT DOES NON-TRADITIONAL MEAN?

If you've been around Soulful Equine for a while you may have
noticed that we often use the word "non-traditional." It's important
that you understand what *we mean* when we use that term, since
there may be variations of it floating around. What does "non-traditional" really mean? Non-traditional, according to the dictionary,
means unconventional; not customary or adhering to accepted
standards.

Let me first give you a little background to our interpretation. I've
noticed there are essentially three groups of people.

The first group believes that anything outside the "norm" can't be
good. People in this group feel norms are established for a reason,
therefore, that's what's best. It's standard practice because it's been
proven over time to work best. This is what has been taught by
people who are considered experts, so they hold it to be true.

The second group of people is at the other end of the spectrum;
anything normal or conventional can't be good. It's the norm because
it's been established by "the establishment." Now this may be true in
some cases. Many powerful and influential people who are part of
the establishment have forced their views upon society in such a way

that those views are now seen as conventional.

This is actually commonplace today. However, it certainly doesn't mean that it's always true. Not every conventional practice has come about that way. Many conventions are accepted standards because they have been proven over and over to work best.

The third group is those people who try to pick and choose what's best from each extreme. They believe extremism in anything is rarely beneficial and realize there's usually something of value to be found in each.

That is the category that Soulful Equine falls into.

*We strive for balance and believe in following the
Hippocratic oath: First do no harm*

We hope to unite these two sides, or at least build a bridge for further discussion, greater learning and helping people to see that something of value can be gleaned from each.

The majority of our beliefs and practices are unconventional, but we always put the well-being of the animal above everything else. We believe in applying the least toxic and least invasive methods. Remember the goal: quality of life and longevity.

FROZEN WITH FEAR

Have you ever heard the saying "Going from 'normal' to 'natural' too quickly can be hazardous to your health"? My version of that saying is:

*Switching from traditional to non-traditional too quickly
can be hazardous to your health.*

Both statements communicate a similar message but in a slightly different context. They're trying to warn you that jumping into some-thing too quickly is not always in your best interest or, in this case, your animal companion's best interest. The intent of these state-ments is to create a feeling inside of you that could help protect you from yourself.

This chapter touches on one word most of us either ignore and/or dread. That one word is something that hides behind excuses when it comes to making important changes in life. This four-letter word is something some of us may hide inside and not feel comfortable discussing with others.

It's the BIG "F" word. FEAR

I'm not here to tell you to ignore your fears and push through them. What I would like to provide here are some strategies you can use when fear seems to get in your way. Each person reacts to fear differently, so it's important to understand how *you* react.

Fear-based decisions are capable of triggering us to do something which results in unnecessary consequences. However, consequences caused by fear can be turned from a negative into a positive. For example, a person who might fear for the health of her family may decide to become more knowledgeable about healthy lifestyles.

Most fear is often subconsciously expressed in the form of procrastination. Don't let fear hold you back, instead, use it as a form of inspiration that causes you to make a change. Don't allow it to paralyze you.

ADDRESSING THE FEAR THAT CAUSES US TO FREEZE

When we feel paralyzed, we're unable to move forward and understand new concepts until we address the underlying issue of fear.. Let's first discuss why fear appears.

Martha Beck is a life coach and author. She did a lot of research on the brain and found that there's a neurological structure that evolved in early vertebrates located in some of the brain's deepest layers. It's wrapped around the cortex of the brain and it sends signals on a regular basis to ensure that we're fed and protected. It's often referred to as the "fight or flight" syndrome. See the Online Resources section for more information on Martha Beck.

When we're afraid, we often have a reaction that causes us to tense up and prepare us to fight, or it prepares us to flee. Horses are this way too, but much more likely to flee than to fight.

What often happens is that people get locked into this intense feeling of anxiety of either fighting or running away. This is what most people do when they become fearful. For example, they're either fighting hard to hold on to what they have or they run away by ignoring what's going on. In the long run, this is not the most productive way to address your fear.

Fear can be a great motivator, and one way to utilize that is to first listen to it. Listen to that voice. Then, take this next step - understand whether or not there's a valid survival mechanism that's underneath it.

Worrying about whether or not your horse is going to hurt you can be a valid fear, especially if at one point you were hurt by your horse. You may have been kicked, bucked off, bitten, etc. What that voice-of-fear tells you is that you have to find ways to gradually increase your confidence around horses. Confidence comes through more knowledge and its practical application. So, you may want to put in the effort to become more knowledgeable about horse behavior and develop the skill to accurately read horses.

Once you examine that fear, you may realize that you never learned how to properly read horses and how to take necessary safety precautions around them. You may not know anything about what it takes to read a horse so you can have fun and stay safe. Therefore, it's understandable that you're going to feel fear.

When you start to identify some of the underlying reasons causing your fears or anxieties, recognize this as a great starting point from which you can move forward and learn.

It's also important in this situation to always protect your confidence. Fear will help you do that, so it's important to listen to it. At the same time, if it's valid, find ways to work through that fear.

WHAT FORM DOES FEAR TAKE?

Fear takes many forms. It can be the fear of rejection, fear of failure, fear of risk, fear of mediocrity, fear of change, self-doubt (which is a form of fear), and the list goes on. Am I fearless? Heck no! In my opinion, no one is completely fearless; it's not in our nature.

The key question is: *How do you manage your fears?* The time fear seems to show up the most is with a risk, a new experience, a learning curve or a challenge of some kind. Let's touch on a few of these areas.

Fear of Mediocrity

I have a close relationship with fear when it comes to mediocrity. I don't want to do something half way or just good enough. This has been something I've battled with throughout my life. How have I finally come to terms with it? Here are a couple of concepts that have helped me:

1) No one is perfect.

I don't believe in doing anything below the standards I have set for myself (which are pretty high), but I finally realized that if I don't let myself off the hook and accept that *no one is perfect* I'll never get anything done or move forward.

No matter what I'm working on or how much I can get done, I won't skimp on quality and will always know that there is room for improvement and growth. I do my best not to allow my fear of mediocrity to get in the way of progress.

2) Take action and accomplish something.

Anything I do, say or write can always be improved upon, but if I don't decide on a cutoff point, I'll never move forward. That almost happened with Soulful Equine. When I finally said, "We need to develop our website and business in stages," I felt great.

It feels fantastic because I've moved in the direction I wanted to go for so many years rather than remaining *frozen and overwhelmed*. Now, I break things down into manageable, bite-sized pieces. I take this approach with most things in my life. Believe me, it's worth it, especially for us over achievers. So the lesson is this: it's important to take action; no one is perfect and it feels great when you accomplish something versus nothing.

Fear of Risk

Humans are uncomfortable when our safety, familiarity and consistency are threatened. *Does this also sound like our friend the Horse?*

No matter how much we accomplish or learn, if we *want to grow* we will continue to venture into new areas that will scare us. There's no way around it. Here are a few concepts that may help you with confronting risk:

1) Take more risk.

Risk-taking can help you to gain more self-confidence through experience. If you don't try something, how will you ever move forward? How will you ever learn and grow?

2) Prepare yourself.

If you prepare yourself ahead of time you'll know what to expect when you step out of your comfort zone. It helps to ask yourself, "What's the worst that could happen?" Usually, it's not all that bad.

3) Just do it.

Sometimes this is a good idea; however, in other situations it may be better to use an approach that helps you gradually overcome your fear of risk. For example, a fear that may need to be gradually overcome is getting on a horse and taking a ride. You may have a huge fear of riding a horse, and you want so badly to make that leap. But in this case it could endanger your life. However, there are ways to help you gradually overcome this fear and feel safe through preparation and confidence building.

Fear is there to keep us safe and is necessary to help us grow and move forward in life. Use fear in a positive manner instead of reacting without thought or preparation. A good rule of thumb to remember is that one fear can build upon another. For example, fear of risk could easily turn into fear of mediocrity. You can move past the fear of risk by preparing yourself so you know what to expect, but then the fear of it not working perfectly causes you to not take action.

Do your best to balance the gift fear gives you and use it to move forward in whatever it is that you want to do.

If you got this far in the chapter you may ask yourself, what does this have to do with horses? It has everything to do with them!

Fear is usually the biggest challenge many people face
when it comes to almost anything related to horses.

If we want to achieve all that we're capable of in life, our challenge is not to overcome fear but rather to influence it, feel it, acknowledge it and then do what we need to do to move forward in spite of it.

Fear survives because we give it a place to exist.

If you don't care about growth, excellence or living life to its fullest then you don't need to worry about fear. It's *traditional* to just settle and to always wonder if it could have been different "if only I had..."

If you do care about moving past your fears in order to live a full life, then do what it takes to manage them. Don't give into your fears - it'll be worth it.

It's important to understand that we are usually our own worst enemy when it comes to dealing with our fears in relation to our horses. Fear is there to both protect us and cause us **to stretch** just enough for us to grow. Be honest with yourself and accept your fear but work on ways to move through it. Do it for your horse and, most of all, for yourself.

Fear of Being Outside the Norm

Embarking upon a direction that is *outside the norm* is intimidating and it's not something that comes naturally for most people. Each person's life experiences are different and valuable in their own way.

When we finally make the decision to change a thought pattern that we have held closely for so long, it can be a challenge and a bit overwhelming. This is why many people choose not to go down the road of change, especially when it's not the traditional way of doing things.

It's called "the road less traveled" for a reason.[3]

How do you *know* if what you choose to embark upon is right for you and your animal companion? You won't know, at least not until you overcome your fear of being outside the norm.

Until that fear is overcome, it will be difficult to be able to faith-

3   M. Scott Peck, The Road Less Traveled: A New Psychology of Love, Traditional Values and Spiritual Growth (New York, NY: Touchstone, 2003)

fully start your discovery process. Once you decide to make a change, you will sometimes get proof immediately that you're on the right track, and other times you'll just have to trust your intuition. What this means is that you may not see the outcome for quite some time.

Intuition is something we must learn to be more aware of and strive to develop, especially when it comes to our horses. Keep in mind, that what usually starts the process of discovery is listening to your intuitive thoughts.

Combining your intuitive thoughts with your logical thoughts can be powerful.

RECLAIM OWNERSHIP OF YOUR OWN MIND AND THOUGHTS

Since I was a toddler, I've had a strong tendency to think for myself. I questioned almost anything that was told to me as well as beliefs that were forced upon me. At that time, I'm sure my parents thought I was just a kid who didn't want to obey, but when I look back on it, this could not have been farther from the truth. I have always had a strong will and a desire to move forward and to grow no matter what others said about my choices.

It's our responsibility to question authority and to reclaim our power to think for ourselves.

THE LEARNING PROCESS

At a very young age, I started having immune system issues. I believe this was a result of the antibiotics my mother gave me anytime I had a sniffle as a child and through my teenage years. That was all she knew at the time and what she was probably taught to do. That belief probably came from her doctor and/or her mother.

I don't fault her, because I believe our parents do the best they can with what they know at the time, as should we. Don't be so hard on yourself or others. Each of us is at a different stage in our lives and in our learning process.

A Journey to Using Non-Traditional Approaches

My journey to being outside the norm started with a strength that enabled me to overcome my fears of ridicule. I have a strong will to question what I'm told. Although this may sound strange, I consider myself fortunate to have had some health problems at a young age.

It gave me the opportunity to turn those problems around and learn from the process. Those experiences helped me have the confidence to learn more about and use non-traditional approaches first on myself, then on my dogs and cats, and finally my horses.

These experiences caused me to be more aware of my intuitive abilities. As I started to use this skill, I began to develop it and put it into practice. There was a lot of study, guidance and application involved.

If I hadn't combined these three processes with my intuition, it would have been more difficult to move through my fears and on to using non-traditional approaches to health care.

It usually takes having to overcome a situation after the experts have failed you. Once something like that happens and you're successful, there's no turning back.

HUMOR AND FEAR

Hmm... humor and fear. What an odd combination. I thought it would be fun to end this section on fear with an exercise. If you'd like to learn more about the humorous side of overcoming your fears, I would recommend the 1991 romantic comedy *Defending Your Life* with Albert Brooks and Meryl Streep. This movie does a great job of addressing the subject of fear.

WHO TO BELIEVE WHEN IT COMES TO HORSE CARE?

"Great minds discuss ideas. Average minds discuss events. Small minds discuss people."
~ Anonymous Proverb

Putting a natural horse care program in place when first starting out can be a challenging task. Like most industries, everyone has an opinion.

I've found that the horse industry is extreme when it comes to most any topic. The extreme aspect usually resides on both sides of the spectrum. Not often do you find opinions that advocate **balance versus extremism**.

Almost anything, no matter how good it is, can be placed into the wrong hands where it's improperly used. News is not about something being great. It's usually about something being wrong and destructive. This is where I feel natural horse care and anything that surrounds it gets the bad end of the deal in many circumstances.

Over the years I have thought long and hard about why so many people have different experiences, both good and bad, when it comes to natural horse care. My conclusion is that these experiences result in everyone forming their opinions about what works and what doesn't.

For example,

> ➤ Metal shoes versus barefoot
> ➤ Traditional equine dentistry versus Natural Balance Dentistry®
> ➤ Use of processed feeds versus whole food form approaches to diet
> ➤ Not using herbs versus using herbal blends
> ➤ Using a bit versus going bitless
> ➤ Keeping horses in stalls versus natural boarding
> ➤ Traditional training methods versus natural horsemanship

I could go on and on with this list. It's no wonder people are so confused, especially when most studies contradict each other and many of them are completely worthless for various reasons.

So, who do you believe? I've asked myself this question for many years and the only answer I've come up with is...

THE HORSE.

When dealing with my own horses and other people's horses in my care, I keep this quote in mind.

> *The trick is not in knowing what to do, rather in knowing when to do it. Everything works sometimes, but nothing works every time. If something fails on even ONE horse, then it must be considered a tool, not a rule!"*
> *~ Cindy Sullivan, Tribe Equus*

Horses are Mother Nature's finest creation and are capable of maintaining a high level of health in the wild; however, man has done a great job of domesticating them and degrading the natural side of the equation. We're great at messing things up and not realizing it. This can cause pain, suffering and illness.

However, there are those who continue to seek answers for their horses. Those are the few individuals who are hopefully not swayed by every popular theory that pops up in the industry.

No one can make you or your horse healthy. With the state of both the human health care industry and the animal care that's available, I believe everyone would be better off by taking charge of their own health and the health of their animal companions.

Knowledge is power; however, beware of whom you obtain your knowledge from. My opinion is that even if a billion people believe something it can still be ridiculous!

I don't take anything that someone says at face value. It doesn't matter to me who they are nor how successful they appear to be. What I have learned over the years is that you must obtain knowledge and take responsibility so you can make informed decisions.

In order to do that, you must first take this important principle to heart: Each horse is **an individual** and you must learn to listen to each *as* an individual.

When learning new concepts, it's important to listen closely to what the horse is asking for at any point in time. What works for one horse may not work for another and, furthermore, it may change from day to day. I've experienced this many times with horses in my care.

That statement alone could indicate why there's so much controversy and confusion about different approaches. Basically, if you want a step-by-step method that always works, there isn't one!

"Adjust to fit the situation." ~ Ray Hunt

The best advice I can give you is to listen closely to your horse.

I can't tell you who or what to believe. You have to figure that out for yourself - it's not an easy journey, but it's an interesting one.

SETTING AN EXAMPLE AND CREATING A MIND SHIFT

Throughout history there have been individuals as well as groups of secret societies who risked their lives because of their beliefs and their strong sense of integrity. In most situations, these people went up against organizations with a lot of power and money. Each of us has certain beliefs that we feel strongly about. A quote that I believe in is:

"Those who stand for nothing, fall for anything."
~ Alex Hamilton

These days you won't hear about people burning at the stake for their beliefs but you will hear constant controversy over certain subjects. It's no different in the horse industry.

For example, there's controversy between approaches to *training* horses versus horse development and forming a close relationship with a horse. You can narrow that down further to traditional horse care versus natural horse care. Then, within the natural horse care community, there's controversy on approaches and even controversy within the natural hoof care community. The list goes on and on, so who do you believe?

It's no wonder most people are confused about horse care. Like you, I've struggled over the years in search of the truth and what's right for my horses. But what does THE TRUTH really mean? All I can say is that no one has all the answers and if someone says she does, I tend to be careful about believing what they say.

Throughout my life, I've come across different extremes of individuals and their approaches (or lack of) to finding answers to their problems.

I'VE OBSERVED THERE ARE THREE CATEGORIES OF PEOPLE

Those who don't want to study or improve themselves and they just need someone to tell them what to do. It may be difficult for them to sift through information and choose an appropriate direction. They usually say... "Just tell me what to do."

Those who study and *want* to improve themselves but they get stuck only believing the teachings of one individual or organization. These people tend to appear "cultish" when it comes to their beliefs and they're closed-minded to other possibilities. This type of individual will usually be pushy with their beliefs and typically scare more people away rather than "converting" them.

Those who seek to continuously improve themselves. This form of improvement starts with personal development. By default, this allows these people to be open to possibilities. At the same time, they stand for something. Usually they take the best from both extremes. They observe, remember and compare. This type of individual wants to be a master at what they do; not a perfectionist or an expert, but a master. Setting good examples comes naturally to them.

> *The result... they plant a seed, they cause a ripple effect*
> *and they create a mind shift.*

I believe that each of us fits into at least one of these categories or a variation there-of. It's part of evolving as an individual. So, what does this have to do with horses? **Everything!**

SIX WAYS TO TELL YOU NEED A NATURAL HORSE CARE COACH

Putting a natural horse care program in place can feel a little overwhelming in the beginning; however, in the long run, it can end up simplifying your horse keeping practices, as well as saving time and money along the way. The biggest benefit is a healthier, happier horse that is *thriving* versus just surviving in domestication.

Hiring someone to help you with your horse care practices may seem strange, but knowing some of the reasons people seek help may cause you to think differently.

Taking that first step to begin something new can be scary. When it comes to subjects such as being a first time horse guardian, taking charge of your horse's care, switching from a traditional to a natural horse care mindset, or learning more about horse behavior, might feel especially scary.

Sometimes there are days you may feel confident about your decisions and other days you might feel confused. It can easily happen when we're too close to the situation and there are times we don't see what is right in front of us. It can be difficult to sift through the mounds of information from friends, TV shows, Internet websites, etc.

> *It's possible to be so overwhelmed with information that*
> *you can become stuck in a pattern where you cause no*
> *change or you create undesirable change.*

Sometimes we need an extra person in the equation who's *been there, done that*, to help us out. Someone who can help us interrupt the pattern of being stuck or confused.

It's easy to think that you're alone in your decision and there's no one who can help you, or maybe you don't want to tell anyone about a decision you've made. You're not the first person who has ever been in a situation where you've wanted to make a leap and cause change when it comes to your horse's care and well-being.

> *Asking for help is not a sign of weakness, it's a sign of strength and intelligence... smart people hire other smart people to help them because they know they can avoid mistakes and reach their goals faster.*

I like to refer to those important people in my life as my "board of directors," so to speak.

But how do you know it's the right time to seek that help and insight when it comes to horses? It doesn't matter if you're just getting started with horses or if you want to start a natural horse care program - the same principles will apply.

There are six ways to tell that you need a natural horse care coach:

1) **You're just getting started with horses** and you want to go down the best and most affordable path possible from a horse care and safety standpoint.

2) **You've been following a traditional horse care program for many years**, but you don't know how to begin a transition to a natural horse care program.

3) **You're using a traditional horse care program**, spending a lot of money and not getting answers or results.

4) **You want to save money with your horse care**, but you can't figure out how to modify your current program to achieve that.

5) **You want to set up a natural boarding arrangement** that will save you time, space, money and improve the health of your horse.

6) **You want to transition your horse from metal shoes to barefoot,** but you don't know if it's right for you or your horse's

situation.

By no means is this an exhaustive list, but it should help you when making the decision to hire a natural horse care coach. Let's look at each point in more detail.

1) You're just getting started with horses.

Being a horse guardian is a huge responsibility. I personally take this responsibility seriously. My belief is that I must be sure about the decision I make because I consider my horses part of my family (the good kind of family). What that means to me is that they're with me for life and if you follow the programs put in place by Soulful Equine, your horse could easily live a happy and healthy life well into her 30s or 40s.

If you're someone who is either purchasing a horse for the first time or you're getting back into horses after many years, you fall into this category. Most people in this category, as a general rule, make big mistakes when purchasing a horse. It's important to consider all that's involved when making this decision.

Going into horse guardianship blindly or with bad advice can cost you not only a large amount of money in the long run but also a lot of fear and frustration. The end result could be that your dream of having a horse could become a nightmare.

I'm sad every time I hear such stories because it's not just the person who suffers but, most of all, the poor horse who was put into the situation. It's important to do your best to avoid such outcomes and hire someone who can help you before you make the leap.

2) You've been following a traditional horse care program for many years, but you don't know how to begin a transition to a natural horse care program.

If traditional horse care has failed you in some way and you want to make a change, you fall into this category. The biggest hurdle I see with individuals in this situation is that they've already gotten a lot of bad advice about starting a natural horse care program or they have difficulty letting go of certain traditional beliefs.

This can result in frustration and confusion and cause you to feel overwhelmed. It can be difficult to intelligently sift through the mounds of information especially when much of it may be half-truths. Finding ways to gradually change old beliefs and, at the same time, not feel overwhelmed, helps to make the transition from normal to natural much smoother.

3) You're using a traditional horse care program, spending a lot of money and not getting answers or results.

I have heard countless stories where traditional horse care practices have failed people and their horses. In many of those situations, individuals spent a lot of money with little or no results and were struggling with the only other option they felt was available, putting the horse down. This is an occurrence that happens more often than most people realize. In many of these situations, traditional care has failed them and their horses.

4) You want to save money with your horse care, but you can't figure out how to modify your current program to achieve that.

There are many unnecessary things that horse guardians spend money on daily that could potentially be cut out. Starting a natural horse care program, by default, will help you save money.

5) You want to set up a natural boarding arrangement.

Some people may think of natural boarding as kicking horses out of the stalls and into a pasture. There is much more to it than that. Although that's one way, it's not the optimal way. The optimal way will help you save time, space, money, and help improve the health of your horse.

6) You want to transition your horse from metal shoes to barefoot.

Many people are on the "barefoot bandwagon" and they think it's easy. They've read an article in a big publication that says anyone can trim their own horses and all you have to do is pull the shoes, do a barefoot trim and it'll work.

I hate to tell you, but there's much more to it. Those statements above are exactly why many people still say that horses can't be sound if they're barefoot and live up to the demands of the domestic-ated horse. Seeking out proper guidance in this area is critical. I can't stress this enough. Hoof care is one of the highest priorities on my horse care list because without a sound horse... well I think you get my drift.

TREATING SYMPTOMS DOESN'T FIX THE PROBLEM

Something to consider that I would like to hit home with is that the items listed here are not real problems. These are actually symp-toms. The problems lie deeper and must be uncovered. Most advice about horse care will usually address only the symptoms of a particu-lar problem.

Speaking with a natural horse care coach one-on-one can help you get to the root of the true problem and help you create a plan to address it. Having a conversation with another human being who knows how to work through this process gives you breakthroughs no book, magazine or online article can ever match. I hope you will make the leap and seek out help when needed.

Something to think about: when equating time with money, less is often more.

Most of us have been there and done that when it comes to spending money unnecessarily. If we'd only had certain information sooner, that could have been avoided. Seeking out advice may also help you get out of an undesirable situation and/or help keep both you and your horse safe and healthy.

THE NATURALLY HEALTHY HORSE CONCEPT

"The way to get started is to quit talking and begin doing." ~ Walt Disney

This chapter will discuss the basics on what you need to consider in order to have a naturally healthy horse. It will give you important concepts necessary for setting up a situation that's relevant to preventing health issues in your horse and that will save you money in the long run.

The lessons in this chapter are simple, but they take time to digest. If you already have some regimented traditional horse care system, you're probably similar to most other horse people out there who have been misinformed. In case no one has informed you yet, that's possibly one of the worst things that could happen to your horse.

A NATURALLY HEALTHY HORSE

Why should you care about the concept of a naturally healthy horse? That's the first question that may go through your mind when you hear the words natural horse care. The short answer is, "You don't have to care."

If you're not concerned about decreased vet bills, less likelihood of disease, decreased or non-existent lameness issues, as well as quality of life and longevity, then there's no reason to care.

Usually the majority of people are short-sighted when it comes to health, not only for themselves but also for the animals in their care. This is a trend, especially in America.

Quick fixes and covering up symptoms is the norm.

Many times it's not so much that they don't care, it's that prevention may not have crossed their mind; it's not on their priority list, or maybe they've been misinformed.

Something to consider is that most likely the "norm" is not in your horse's best interest. So, how do you turn that way of thinking around? I know it's tough and it takes time. As I discussed in the chapters on fear, change is difficult for most people; however, if the change is for the betterment of your horse's health, then why not?

How about creating a mind shift? That mind shift can be pointed toward prevention versus disease. It can be about addressing the underlying cause versus covering up symptoms. By changing those two thought patterns, you'll be well on your way to discovering the secret to quality of life and longevity for both yourself and your horse.

Okay, back to the concept of what a naturally healthy horse is. A naturally healthy horse is not necessarily a horse that never has health issues. However, it is a horse that may rarely have issues. And when something does arise, it's less detrimental than for a horse that is not kept naturally.

For example, take two different horses that are the same age, one is kept naturally and the other is kept traditionally. One day a drastic drop in barometric pressure occurs.

The traditionally kept horse colics and requires colic surgery due to impaction. The naturally kept horse, who had colic issues before being kept naturally, had a spasmodic colic. This horse was helped using a more natural approach, and she was fine. No drugs were needed to help her through her colic episode, even though a veterinarian was called as a precautionary measure.

Basically, both horses had a colic episode because there was some other underlying problem. Just because the one horse was kept naturally does not mean she may not have health issues on occasion.

The point is that unlike the traditionally kept horse, the naturally kept horse was more likely to live through the colic episode and its treatment did not require an expensive vet bill.

FULL ENGAGEMENT

A naturally healthy horse is fully engaged. Full engagement requires four related but separate sources of energy.

These sources include, physical, emotional, and mental as well as spiritual.

Yes, I'm adding the spiritual in there, too. All four are important to a healthy horse. If all four of these areas are managed effectively you can have a naturally healthy horse AND achieve your goals. It's important to focus on exactly how you can effectively manage those areas of your horse's life so you can get the results you want.

No matter what kind of horse regimen you're on, you will want to continue learning and figuring out what's best for both your situation and your horse. First, you must start with an open mind and a willingness to learn.

HORSE HEALTH – TRUTH REVEALED

Before expressing my thoughts on the truth about current day horse health, I would like to share a quote you may like that's bold but true:

"Sometimes common sense trumps empirical evidence."
~ Dr. Joseph Mercola

What does "healthy as a horse" really mean? If you want a healthy horse, the answer goes back to the subject of *who do you believe*?

Just imagine yourself in a situation, like Scrooge, in the story *A Christmas Carol*, by Charles Dickens. No, I don't mean to imagine being *like* Scrooge (in the beginning he was not very kind), but imagine you have the ability to see the past, present and future when it comes to horse health; and so your journey begins.

HORSE HEALTH – THE PAST

Your first stop is in the past, and you find yourself watching our noble friends, the wild horses, in their most healthy state - roaming freely. Their soundness is beyond anything you've seen in domestication as they float across the terrain, seamlessly feeling the ground under their bare hooves with every beat.

Their highly structured society demonstrates their need for interaction as they play, compete for dominance and rest in the sun. Their beauty and healthy state takes your breath away. You've never seen anything like it.

HORSE HEALTH - THE PRESENT

Your next stop is in the present. You suddenly realize you're at one of the Bureau of Land Management (BLM) holding facilities and you notice groups of horses that once roamed freely now standing in enclosed quarters with limited movement.

You approach the pens to get a closer look. What you see is astonishing. The once beautifully shaped sound hooves are now overgrown and chipping away. Those wild horses that once floated seamlessly across the terrain are now at a standstill.

As you sadly look on, you note something is missing and you have trouble putting a finger on it. Then you realize the **spirit** *and* **dignity** that once radiated off these magnificent creatures is gone.

Some of the horses have become ill from the BLM round ups and some have even died. How could this be? How can we take something so healthy, strong and vibrant and mess it up so badly? You can't stand to watch anymore so you decide to move on to the future hoping that something has changed - surely someone has done something to help these horses.

You keep thinking that someone has to step in before these beautiful free-roaming animals become extinct. After all, these wild horses are a symbol of our American heritage and freedom.

HORSE HEALTH - THE FUTURE

Thankfully, you step into the future, only to find yourself faced with a grim reality. Not only are the wild horses extinct, but our domestic-ated horses are experiencing more health problems than ever before. We no longer have a way of truly knowing how the wild horse stayed so healthy for so long without human interference. Our treasured wild horse models are gone.

THE TRUTH

Back to the current day and what is happening with our horses. What is the truth about our horses' health? Unfortunately, our horses today are sicker than ever before. As we continue to address symp-toms, causes are often overlooked. As we ignore Mother Nature, intuition and common sense, and instead focus on statistics and studies, our horses suffer. The wild horse is nature's finest creature. We should treasure it and learn everything we can from it. *That's* the truth revealed.

HOW DOES THIS APPLY TO YOUR HORSE'S HEALTH?

Is it about saving the wild horses? Is it about humans doing unneces-sary things **to** horses in order to keep them "healthy," while unknowingly causing them to become more and more unhealthy? Is it about the human needing to accept that sometimes common sense really *does* trump empirical evidence?

PROTECTING THE WILD HORSE – A SYMBOL OF OUR AMERICAN HERITAGE

There has been a lot in the press on the massive round-ups of our country's wild horses by the Bureau of Land Management (BLM). When I say *massive*, I'm not exaggerating. As of 2010, these have been the largest roundups of wild horses in history.

All you have to do is Google "wild horse roundup" and you'll find plenty of information on it. Most people are unaware of the devastation that has been going on, not to mention how our media choose to interpret truth versus the reality of what is really happening to our wild horse population.

A LITTLE BACKGROUND ON THE WILD HORSE

The history of America's wild, free roaming horses is not common knowledge for most people. Most refer to wild horses as "mustangs." In reality they're basically offspring of domestic horses that have either escaped or been released into the wild. The more correct term is *feral horses*. They're not a special breed of horse, like most people assume.

They're able to survive in some of the harshest desert lands and are healthier than any domestic horses I see on a daily basis. This goes to show that we have much to learn from them and their ability to successfully adapt to a life in the wild where they remain healthy and sound. Horses are extremely adaptable and that's why they have survived for millions of years.

MY PERSONAL REASONS FOR ADDRESSING THIS ISSUE

I have to admit that the term "wild horse," referring to feral horses, never crossed my mind until around 2002. That was the time when I started researching and becoming involved in natural hoof care.

Many of you who have horses probably have had no obvious reas-on to think about the wild horses in our country. Some people probably have no idea that wild horses still exist!

I'm here to inform you that they *do* exist and they're healthy and roaming free. I'm also here to tell you that if you're not thinking about them, now is the time to start.

The wild horse is our model for the optimally healthy horse.

Wild horses hold the answers to teaching us ways of overcoming the multitude of health problems we face with our horses in domestication. Once again, they're a model of beauty, knowledge, and power. They are the most noble of creatures.

Have you ever asked yourself why we use the horse as a symbol for so many things in our country? The answer, in my opinion, is a no-brainer. Horses got us to where we are today. They helped us evolve as *they* have evolved.

They were there to help us when we had to feed our families, when we didn't have tractors to plow our fields, and they were there for us when automobiles didn't exist. They were there for us when the original mailman road his pony to ensure delivery of our mail, which allowed us to communicate with our loved ones across the country, and they were there for us during emergencies when we needed the Cavalry to save us.

During the Great Depression, there was an unlikely champion who became a symbol of hope to many Americans. His name was Seabiscuit, and he was a great thoroughbred, racehorse champion. I believe Seabiscuit played a huge role in reminding us that there is hope and that the underdog *can* succeed. Again, THE HORSE is a symbol of our American heritage.

WHY SHOULD YOU BE CONCERNED?

This is not the first time there has been a public outcry over the inhumane treatment of wild horses during roundups and removal. Congress passed two laws to help protect America's wild horses.

In 1959, Public Law 86-234, known as the Wild Horse Annie Act, was passed. It prohibited the inhumane methods used to destroy and capture wild horses.

In 1971, Public Law 92-195, the <u>Wild Free-Roaming Horse and Burro Act</u>, was passed. This was a much more comprehensive law. In short, it gave responsibility for the protection and management of the wild horses and burros to the BLM.

The "Congressional findings and declaration of policy" from this act states:

> *"Congress finds and declares that wild free-roaming horses and burros are living symbols of the historic and pioneer spirit of the West; that they contribute to the diversity of life forms within the Nation and enrich the lives of the American people; and that these horses and burros are fast disappearing from the American scene. It is the policy of Congress that wild free-roaming horses and burros shall be protected from capture, branding, harassment, or death; and to accomplish this they are to be considered in the area where presently found, as an integral part of the natural system of the public lands."*

I would like to make it clear that it's important that our wild horse populations are managed but in a humane manner and without deception. The problem with these laws, like so many in the United States, is that they're rarely enforced, or unjustly enforced.

Most of the BLM round-ups that are going on are cruel and brutal, and many of these beautiful icons of our American Heritage are losing their lives.

The BLM *continues to violate* the 1971 protection act. Not only that, but our taxpayer dollars are being spent on this project.

As a citizen and an animal lover, it's important to be concerned!

> *"I believe, as do so many of my fellow Americans, that the wild horse is an irreplaceable national treasure. It would be a tragic mistake to allow this noble creature to disappear from our western landscape."* ~ Robert Redford

I hope this information has prompted you to take action in helping to protect our wild horses.

COMMON HEALTH CONCERNS FOR HORSE GUARDIANS

"The doctor of the future will give no medicine, but will instruct his patient in the care of the human frame, in diet and in the cause and prevention of disease."
~ Thomas A. Edison

Understanding the importance of prevention is the first step in helping your horse thrive. Most common health problems plaguing our domesticated horses can be minimized, if not completely eliminated, by implementing key natural horse care concepts.

As I've already discussed, most of what you may currently believe or have been taught about horse care is most likely not in your horse's best interested. This chapter covers important concepts for you to understand that will help you be aware of horse care approaches that can cause many common health concerns. These traditional approaches to horse care are not only detrimental but are also unnecessary.

PARASITE RESISTANCE IN HORSES AND CHEMICAL DEWORMING

As a horse guardian, it's important that you manage the worm burden of your horse; that is, if there actually is one. Traditional approaches to addressing parasites in horses has caused a serious concern called *parasite resistance*.

Parasite resistance in horses has been an ongoing problem for many years. The concern, which is a valid one, is that we're creating "super" bugs and that it's only a matter of time before nothing works. One of the main causes of this problem is the unnecessary and over-use of chemical dewormers.

The average horse guardian may not be aware of the impact this particular problem is beginning to have on the horse industry. Although some of the first reports of resistance to deworming drugs date back to the early 1960s, it has now become an even greater concern. This concern over parasite resistance is actually growing worldwide and is not something to be taken lightly.

DENMARK'S APPROACH TO PARASITES IN HORSES

I came across an interesting article called *Parasites in Horses: Are You Playing Your Part?* on Horsetalk.co.nz. I discovered that in 1999, Denmark enforced a law where horse guardians could no longer purchase chemical dewormers (called "drenches" in some countries) over the counter.

This came about because of the growing concern over resistance issues. Many horse guardians are using dewormers inappropriately, which is causing a rapid growth of parasite resistance to these drugs.

Denmark's solution to this problem was to take it out of the hands of the horse guardian and make it a prescription only drug. It placed worm control into the hands of the veterinarians, who have to be satisfied that a horse's worm burden is great enough to require chemical deworming. There may come a time, as it has in Denmark, when we can no longer purchase over the counter dewormers in the United States. I believe there are pros and cons to that decision.

PARASITE RESISTANCE NEEDS TO BE TAKEN SERIOUSLY

The intent of this section is to shed light on the growing issue of parasite resistance and to stress that it needs to be taken seriously. Parasitologists agree that horse guardians need to have a strategy for deworming including monitoring the long term effectiveness of their programs, which can be done using fecal egg counts. This will give the guardian an overall picture of whether or not their horse needs to be chemically dewormed.

Rotating chemical dewormers is no longer the answer to the worm resistance problem that has been created.

The misconception is that all horses have to be treated for worms.

Something that is becoming more common is checking your horse for worms *first*, rather than blindly deworming them without knowing their worm burden. All horses are exposed to worms but not all have worms or, if they do, the worm burden may be minimal and manageable by the horse.

If we do fecal exams and only treat our horses if they need it, then we're contributing to the overall health of our horses as well as minimizing the amount of chemicals we put into our environment. We're also minimizing our contribution to the worm resistance problem.

Completely eliminating parasites in our horses is not realistic, but by conducting fecal egg counts you can build a picture of each horse's sensitivity to parasites and determine the effectiveness of the program you have in place. That program may be either a chemical or a wholistic program, and some people use a combination of the two.

No matter what the program, it's important to know if it's working.

No chemical dewormer is 100% effective; therefore, it's important to check your horse by doing a fecal egg count and *not* to treat all your horses the same. You must tailor a program to each individual horse.

A big misconception is that if one horse in the herd has a high worm burden, then all the horses in that herd must be infested. I can tell you for a fact, that is not a true statement, and I have witnessed it in my own herd. Therefore, be sure not to give into the peer pressure of deworming all your horses just because **one** *might* need it.

Keep in mind that you're part of the resistance problem every time you make the decision to chemically deworm your horse.

If treatment is necessary, the range of time between each treatment can vary. Sometimes treatment is not needed at all. What's appropriate for one farm or horse may not apply to another. Patterns of resistance can vary from country to country, state to state, and even between properties. Many guardians simply decide to stick to a routine of chemically deworming their horses without using fecal egg count tests. This is the mentality that continues to contribute to the problem of parasite resistance.

This mindset may also put horses at risk who don't need drugs to fight off parasites. They may already have their own natural resistance built up.

Have you ever thought about how wild horses control parasites? As far as I know, they're not getting chemically dewormed every six weeks.

SAY GOODBYE TO OLD DEWORMING STANDARDS

Although it's been drilled into our heads that we should chemically deworm our horse every 6-8 weeks, it's time to say goodbye to that approach. This is an old way of thinking that needs to change.

What if your horse didn't have a worm burden and you still gave her a chemical dewormer every 6-8 weeks? Do you think it's wise to continue to give her chemicals when it's not needed?

When it comes to your horse's overall well-being and longevity, the wholistically minded individual understands that it's unnecessary and irresponsible, not to mention how harmful it is to the environment.

YOUR BEST DEFENSE

Most sports have a saying that "your best defense is a strong offense." The offense I use in the war on parasites is a GREAT immune system.

A great immune system starts in the digestive system. Therefore, you must have a healthy digestive system in order to have a great immune system. The funny thing about that is the more you chemically deworm your horses, the more you're compromising both the digestive and the immune system.

A naturally kept horse's immune system is usually much stronger than a more traditionally kept horse. By default, the majority of traditionally kept horses have an immune system that's already taxed.

You may think that your horse doesn't have issues; however, if you have to deworm her every 6-8 weeks since she doesn't have her own resistance built up, then that is an issue with the immune system as well as your horse keeping practices.

> *"The message I would like to stress is that a healthy immune system is important when it comes to keeping the numbers of internal parasites low." ~ Stephanie Krahl*

USING FECAL EGG COUNT RANGES AS A GUIDELINE

Fecal egg counts will determine the number of eggs per gram (EPG) in the manure. This eggs-per-gram number is a standard measure and, depending on the number, it will determine if your horse is carrying a low, moderate or high worm burden. Keep in mind as you're reading these values that it's not necessary to maintain a zero fecal egg count.

There are no hard and fast rules, and you will run into differing opinions, but below are some general guidelines I use when determining the extent of the worm burden in a horse:

➢ Unimportant (50 EPG or less)
➢ Low (75 - 225 EPG)
➢ Moderate (250 - 650 EPG)
➢ High (650+ EPG)

(Note that EPG is determined by taking the number of eggs found and multiplying by 25.)

Some companies that do fecal egg counts recommend chemically deworming at levels I consider low. The low to moderate burden could more than likely be addressed by boosting the immune system and giving the horse the support she needs in order to manage the minimal parasite load.

Again, every horse is different. Some may have a count considered moderate to high, but show no signs whatsoever, including common related issues such as digestive upset (i.e. colic), poor hoof quality or a dull coat. This demonstrates that the horse is more than likely able to manage the worm burden.

You have to be careful to use your best judgment.

Every horse and every situation is different, so please use these numbers **as a guide, not as a rule**.

Something else to throw into the mix, think about horses that initially arrive at a rescue facility. Their health is usually significantly compromised. They may be heavily infested with parasites and demonstrate all the common signs of a high worm burden, but if they were to be chemically dewormed without being allowed to first regain their health, it's possible they would have an adverse reaction to such a sudden purging.

This is just one example. Please keep in mind that if a horse does have a high worm count, it may be best to proceed with caution in using a chemical dewormer, because it's possible that an issue, such as colic, could be induced.

MY RULE OF THUMB

I always ask myself this question before I take any kind of action with my horses, "Will the action I'm about to take compromise my horse's immune system?" If the answer is yes, I'll do my best to find an alternative. If there's not an alternative that works, then I do everything I can to find a way to minimize compromising the immune system or I give them extra nutritional support during those times of stress.

Just for the record, the list of items below (and this is not a complete list) can compromise a horse's immune system and leave them more open to disease:

➤ Over vaccinating
➤ Use of chemical dewormers
➤ Use of chemical fly sprays
➤ Stress during travel or change in environment
➤ Any feed or hay produced using any kind of chemical
➤ Processed feeds
➤ Diets high in starch and sugar

FIGHTING WORM RESISTANCE: WHAT TO CONSIDER

Below is a list of items to consider when it comes to fighting worm resistance:

➤ Check your horses for parasites regularly using fecal egg counts.
➤ The misconception is that all horses have worms so we continue to deworm without knowing our horse's worm burden, that is, if they have one.
➤ Rotating chemical dewormers is no longer the answer to the worm resistance problem that's been created.
➤ All horses are exposed to worms, but the worm burden may be minimal.
➤ Using chemical dewormers on a regular 6-8 week schedule could be harming your horse (even more than the worms themselves) by weakening her immune system and her natural resistance against them.
➤ Use of chemical dewormers may also contribute to laminitis.
➤ Horse keeping programs that chemically deworm often, no matter if they have a worm burden or not, are contributing to the worm resistance issues existing today.
➤ To minimize exposure to parasites, put paddock management techniques in place.

FLY CONTROL FOR HORSES, A NON-TOXIC PROGRAM

At Soulful Equine, we believe in non-toxic approaches to almost anything we do when it comes to our horses, pets and our health. As I stated in the section on *Parasite Resistance in Horses and Chemical Deworming*, you must pay close attention to anything that could compromise your horse's immune system.

Heavy usage of toxic chemicals for fly control is not only unnecessary but is also harmful to your horse's health and to yours. It also contributes to the environmental issues of over-using chemicals.

Whenever it's within our control to use or not use toxic chemicals, we should not use them.

Keep in mind that you encounter large numbers of toxins in your environment just by breathing and being alive. However, anytime you have the opportunity to minimize the effect it has on your horses and you, you should *take that responsibility seriously*. See our Online Resources section for more information on ways to manage flies in a non-toxic manner.

FLY SPRAYS

If at all possible, use fly sprays that are approved for use on certified organic farms or make your own. I look for fly sprays that are non-toxic, effective, and don't leave a greasy residue. I've tested many different "natural" fly sprays and still go back to the ones you can find through our Online Resources section of this book.

GARLIC FOR HORSES

In the section on *Fly Control for Horses, A Non-Toxic Program*, I discussed the importance of using methods that reduce, if not eliminate, the number of toxic chemicals used when controlling flies. The section on fly control is not complete without talking about *garlic*.

I want to provide a little direction when it comes to using garlic, especially for helping to control both internal and external pests. For more information on parasite control, see the section in this book on *Parasite Resistance in Horses and Chemical Deworming*.

If you Google "horses and garlic" you will get a significant amount of information on the subject, so I'm going to stick to what my own personal beliefs and experiences have been when it comes to using this wonderful herb.

A General Overview

Garlic is the best-known and most widely used herb in the horse world and for good reason. It's one of those substances that Mother Nature provides that can assist us in many situations. It's rich in natural sulfur, and can sometimes help in reducing internal parasites. It helps to cleanse the blood and, when excreted, will help with repelling external pests, such as biting flies or ticks.

Garlic is a natural antibiotic. It's especially ideal for almost any respiratory problem, which I personally experienced with one of my horses many years ago. Since it is both an antibiotic and it assists in soothing a cough, it can help with mucus in the lungs and any infection that's present.

Another attribute of garlic is its ability to improve digestion by supporting the development of natural bacterial flora. This is the key to a good digestive system which, in-turn, is important to a strong immune system. If you'd like to help protect yourself and your animals from infection, this is one of the best herbs to turn to.

My Personal Experiences with Garlic

Now that you have the CliffsNotes version of some of garlic's benefits, I'll share with you my personal experiences and thoughts about using this herb for horses. First of all, I tend to liken garlic to apple cider vinegar. They're both capable of so much natural healing, but the results will vary depending on how your or your horse's body prioritizes the issue needing help first.

Both are in the form Mother Nature intended (*whole food, minimal if no processing*) which is one of the reasons they both have so many benefits. Most people might think, "Wow that must be a miracle substance," but in actuality, when the body is given the nutrients it needs in the proper form, the results can be amazing.

I feed garlic to my horses and have used this herb for over a decade on my two oldest horses. I know that the quality of the herb you purchase is important.

Some processing methods will compromise the product, and then you're wasting your money and you end up thinking it doesn't work. Despite the fact that this herb has been used safely and successfully for thousands of years, garlic is starting to get a reputation that it's bad for horses based on supposed scientific information from the veterinarian and equine nutritionist communities.

This is usually the case when something works "too well." This happens often in both the animal and human health industries. I could provide a lot of data and scientific studies showing that vitamin C is bad and causes ill effects. I could also provide many contradicting studies showing how beneficial vitamin C is. Studies that show the benefits are more often results of that substance being provided in its proper form and with all its co-factors. It goes back to processing and quality. I can't stress this enough.

Remember you can find contradicting studies on anything.

On that note, be careful where you purchase your garlic and understand, as best you can, what processing procedures that company uses. Some processing methods, as stated, will compromise the integrity of product ingredients. Remember it's more cost effective for companies to use cheap ingredients and create highly processed food stuff that will have a longer shelf life. This is normally not good for you, your pets or your horse.

Something else to be cautious about; companies will change formulations of their products thinking they're improving them or so they can save money. Both reasons usually result in a product of poor quality or that has ingredients you should avoid feeding to your horse. This has happened to me on multiple occasions. **Always be sure to read the ingredient labels**, even if you've been purchasing that item for a long time. Companies seem to be allowed to change formulations without announcing it, so you have to be observant.

I use straight garlic and it usually comes in granule or powdered form. My horses like both, and it doesn't matter which form I feed to them. Some horses are picky and may not eat one form or the other, so it's best to experiment.

Even quality garlic is not too expensive and **not much is required** when you're feeding it to horses. If your horses don't mind the taste, you may need to bump up the amount you give them during the times of the year when external pests are at their peak. Again, it's best to experiment with the amount and be sure to read the manufacturer's recommendations.

If you do increase the amount during high infestation times, you'll need to allow time for it to build up in the horse's system. Since this is an herb and not a drug, and it works naturally with the body, it's best to give it about two to four weeks to build up in the system.

One More Note on External Pests

Something else worth mentioning that I have noticed over the years, no matter what horse facility I go to, there will be certain horses that *attract* more flies than others. In my experience, this is usually an indicator of a horse who is more compromised (immune system) than the other horse(s) around her.

The level of a horse's pest, fly or parasite attractant can correlate to how healthy they are or to them being fed an unnatural and inappropriate diet.

Don't over analyze this concept; it's good to just be aware of it. A quick example in my own small herd of three is that during the summer months, the flies will usually gravitate over to my more compromised horse - my insulin resistant (IR) challenged horse. All three of my horses can be standing side by side and the flies will almost always gravitate over to him.

COULD DRASTIC CHANGES IN BAROMETRIC PRESSURE AFFECT YOUR HORSE?

During certain times of the year, dramatic weather changes can occur quickly. One day it's beautiful, 71 degrees and sunny, and the next day there's a drastic 40 degree drop in temperature. That happened here in Texas over Christmas in 2009. A drastic drop in the barometric pressure started to occur the day before Christmas Eve. On Christmas Eve day, a blizzard blew in bringing a heavy snow, rain and sleet mix with winds over 45 mph. For a native Texan, it was miserable.

Drastic weather changes can cause problems for both our horses and us. When the barometer drops dramatically just prior to a big storm, some horses, as well as people, can experience ill effects. To my knowledge, there's no documented proof that there's a correlation between weather and physical problems in horses; however, it has been shown that a link exists between barometric pressure and headaches in humans.

For example, some people consistently have a flare up of a physical ailment such as TMJ, knee pain, back pain, headaches and the list can go on. Additionally, we can also be more susceptible to a cold or flu bug. For horses, some may experience mild to severe colic during a sudden barometric pressure drop when a cold front is coming through.

Some people may believe that's a myth, but just for fun give your nearest vet clinic a call the day after a drastic weather change in your area and politely ask if they would share with you how many cases of colic were reported the day of the drop.

One vet clinic I spoke with in the area reported that one of their vets had 4 farm calls for colic and two horses that had to go in for surgery that day. I find this interesting. Just think of how many other vets had similar experiences.

Some people feel that it's due to a lack of water consumption, and that may be true. However, I believe it's not necessarily the barometric drop that causes these types of problems, but rather that it's helping to point out an underlying issue.

Some horses are more sensitive than others to weather changes. Unfortunately, there's not much we can do about this. What we *can* do is to be aware of the possibility and take precautions.

A few ideas:

➢ Keep your horse in a natural environment that allows free movement.

➢ Provide a quality probiotic when you know changes in the weather will be approaching.

➢ If the weather is drastically changing or is about to change, avoid making modifications that might stress the horse in any way including diet, housing, travel or exercise.

➢ Make sure your horse is drinking enough water and is not showing a change in her eating patterns.

➢ Keep a close eye out for any sudden changes in your horse's behavior including symptoms of colic.

➢ Keep a healthy maintenance program in place, and try to eliminate as many other causes of colic that you can.

➢ One of the biggest causes of colic is a high parasite loads. Do fecal checks so you know your horse's parasite load patterns. See the *Parasite Resistance in Horses and Chemical Deworming* section of this book for more information.

This subject may seem like common sense, but it's worth pointing out that there could be a possible correlation between your horse's health and certain weather patterns.

If, Heaven forbid, something does happen to your horse in such a situation, take a closer look at what the underlying cause may be.

The weather was more than likely the "straw that broke the camel's back," so to speak, and may be a warning of an underlying problem that was possibly overlooked.

THE DREADED WORD - COLIC

Colic is one of those things in the horse world that can be serious and result in the death of your horse. I believe its occurrence is too common. By following the core principles of keeping a naturally healthy horse, this dreaded situation can become much less of a concern.

Like nutrition, colic is a fairly large subject to cover in a short section of a book. The combination of the subjects, colic and natural horse care, can almost be a book in itself. For more information on colic please see our Online Resource section of the book.

Before I go much further, what is colic in horses? Colic is basically abdominal pain. You may think, why all the fuss? It's just a stomachache. In horses, it can be much more. The abdominal pain the horse experiences is not a diagnosis, rather it's a clinical sign. The word "colic" is a catch all for the different forms of gastrointestinal issues a horse can encounter.

If your horse experiences colic, the episode can range from fairly minor in nature to your horse requiring emergency surgery. Colic surgery is an expensive procedure and like all surgeries, no matter how routine, there's always the possibility that your horse won't make it through the surgery.

Colic is the **leading** cause of death in horses, with laminitis being a close second. The more you learn about natural horse care, the more you'll come to realize that these two leading causes of death are closely related. I believe they both have the same underlying cause: unnatural and inappropriate horse keeping practices. I look at the underlying cause of colic the same way I do laminitis when it comes to horse care.

Although this is not *proven*, horses kept naturally are less likely to have a colic episode and if they do, more than likely it will be minor. As a naturally minded individual, since you know that colic has to do with the digestive system, maybe it's a good idea that you do everything you can not to compromise it. This is one approach.

Let's look at some unnatural horse keeping practices that compromise the health of the horse.

UNNATURAL HORSE KEEPING PRACTICES

Infrequent feedings

Only feeding your horse 2-3 times per day can cause digestive upset and lead to ulcers. Mother Nature intended for horses to forage continuously, meaning, they're able to move freely and seek out their food - they're not restricted. Most horse guardians do the complete opposite by restricting meals and not allowing the horse continuous movement.

Horses are designed much differently than we are. They produce gastric acid continuously and for good reason. They're designed to eat constantly.

Feeding your horse properly is a huge subject to cover, but I want to make it clear that what I stated here doesn't mean you should feed your horse free choice grain and/or legume hay, i.e. alfalfa or clover. Rather, it's appropriate to feed free choice **grass hay** which needs to be low in sugar, starch and fructan (collectively known as Non Structural Carbohydrates NSC).

Not providing good foundational nutrition

Most horse guardians do not provide good foundational nutrition. I cover that subject in detail in this book. Without a good foundation in place, you're asking for problems.

Over feeding grain or feeding processed commercial feeds

Despite popular belief, horses do not need grain. If you do feed grain, you can feed a small amount of it to provide some variety. It's best to avoid processed feeds and to create your own mix. This is one way to help keep your horse safe so you don't have to worry about that next feed recall.

Not incorporating a good dental program into your horse keeping practices

We haven't addressed dental care in this book, but it's an extremely important part of keeping your horse healthy, sound and balanced. A big problem I see is that most people rely on their veterinarian to take care of their horse's dental work, or they don't address the horse's dental needs at all.

All I can say to that is, "*Would you allow your general practitioner doctor to do YOUR dental work?*" I bet the answer to that question is no. Remember that not all equine dentists are the same.
I use Natural Balance Dentistry® and have since 2006.

> **Equine dentistry isn't necessarily just about eating and digestion, it's even more so about neurological function, body mass, soundness and balance.**

I would highly recommend you learn more about *Natural Balance Dentistry®* and avoid using veterinarians and *traditional* equine dentists for your horse's dental work. You can find more information about equine dentistry in our Online Resources section.

Not allowing your horse to eat at ground level

Horses were not meant to eat from hay and grain feeders raised off the ground. It's important for the health of your horse's digestive system to feed them at ground level. Allowing your horse to eat at ground level is also important to help prevent some of the more common dental problems in horses, which could result in less dental work.

Not enough movement

I cover the subject of movement extensively throughout this book. Limited movement is another unnatural horse keeping practice. By default, if a horse gets plenty of movement it can assist the digestive system in working more effectively. Some professionals (and I'm one of them) believe that plenty of movement is thought to reduce the incidence of colic. However, people on the other side of the fence say it *hasn't been proven*. To that I would say, once again, "Sometimes common sense trumps empirical evidence."

Excessive use of chemical dewormers

Chemical dewormers will not only kill off all the bad guys, but they can also kill off the good bacteria in the digestive system. Another important point to note is if your horse is heavily infested, and you chemically deworm her, you could cause a quick die-off of the parasites and basically induce colic in your horse. If your horse is infested with parasites, there's another underlying problem that needs to be addressed.

A Higher Likelihood of Colic

By no means is this an exhaustive list of ways that can help prevent colic. The point I wanted to stress is that *unnatural horse keeping practices* can result in a higher likelihood of colic.

SIGNS THAT YOUR HORSE IS HAVING A COLIC EPISODE

I would like to point out that it's important to be aware of what's normal for **your horse** and what's abnormal. This will come in handy when you're reading over some of the clinical signs of colic. When trying to determine if your horse is actually having a colic episode, it may help to think how you would feel if you had severe abdominal pains.

Below is a list of some of the signs of colic:

➢ Excessive pacing
➢ Stretching like she's uncomfortable in the abdominal area
➢ Pawing
➢ Looking back excessively or biting at the flank/stomach area
➢ Lying down, rolling and getting back up excessively
➢ Making groaning sounds like she's in pain
➢ Loss of appetite combined with some of the other symptoms
➢ Trouble urinating
➢ Decreased manure output
➢ Increased pulse rate
➢ No sounds from the stomach

You're basically looking for abnormal behavior from your horse. It's important to always call your veterinarian if you suspect colic.

WHILE WAITING ON YOUR VETERINARIAN

While waiting on your veterinarian, here's a brief list of some things you can do to help your horse:

- ➤ If your horse wants to lie down, don't allow it. She could cause the intestinal tract to twist with excessive rolling.
- ➤ Do not force your horse to walk. If she wants to walk, gently move with her while you have her in hand (haltered).
- ➤ Some people use specific homeopathy remedies during this time. This subject is beyond the scope of this book, but I'll provide other educational materials in the Online Resources section.
- ➤ I have personally used Photonic therapy (red light therapy) and Equine Touch to stop a spasmodic colic in a horse. Usually you can stop the colic before the veterinarian arrives. This is not always the case, so be sure to call your veterinarian first.

In any situation that pertains to an emergency with your horse, the better your relationship, the more willing a partner she will be during a traumatic situation despite her fear.

I have witnessed this on more than one occasion and have talked with other equine guardians on the subject. It's amazing because your horse knows you're trying to help them and they'll work with you, not against you.

Be sure to prepare now. Don't wait until something happens. If you have developed a strong bond with your horse, it will show, and those traumatic situations will, more than likely, result in a good ending with no struggle.

I hope this section has shed a slightly different light on the subject of colic and the importance of keeping a naturally healthy horse. For further reading about colic, please see the Online Resources section of this book.

TO BLANKET YOUR HORSE OR NOT TO BLANKET... THAT IS THE QUESTION

Have you ever thought about why people blanket their horses in the winter? If you question and explore this practice, you may be surprised by what you'll learn. Blanketing horses in the winter is a common horse keeping practice when it starts to get a little chilly outside. Yes, you heard me right, a *little chilly*.

During the first onset of colder weather, I notice many horses with their flashy blankets on. Since I live in the middle of one of the larger horse areas in the country, I don't have to drive far before I spot one or two horses like this.

IS YOUR HORSE REALLY COLD?

Horses are masters at regulating their own body temperature. It's easy for you to get in the way of what Mother Nature intended by blanketing your horse and or keeping her in a heated barn. It's also easy to take human thoughts and actions and apply them to your horse. This is when we get ourselves into trouble and our horse keeping practices become inferior and detrimental.

Most people think that their horse will get cold and that she needs a nice, cushy stall to bed down in each night. This kind of thinking only makes the human feel better. This is a human thought and action that's applied to horses versus thinking like a horse and understanding a horse's true nature.

As I mentioned earlier in this chapter, we had a blizzard in Texas on Christmas Eve day in the winter of 2009. Yes, a blizzard in Texas. The barometric pressure dropped quickly and we had strong wind gusts of over 45 mph. Two of my horses are in their mid-twenties. One of them is the horse that got me into natural hoof care when he got laminitis. Each year I allow my horses to grow their natural winter coats. They were outside during that storm and they were *not blanketed*.

They have wonderful wind blocks provided by my barn as well as multiple shelters. They're always able to get out of the elements on their own. There are no stalls and I don't waste my money on shavings. I also don't bother spending money on expensive blankets.

All a horse needs is a shelter and wind blocks (not a stall) so they can get out of the *extreme elements* if they choose. Notice I said extreme elements. They don't need a stall bedded deep with shavings, and they don't need a blanket or a warm barn.

A horse blanket can impair the circulation around the shoulder area creating tension in the neck, which can cause discomfort or other physical problems. This can also happen if the blanket is left on for long periods of time, even if it fits properly.

So why spend extra money on either?

Think how much you can save over time on shavings alone. Just for a minute, think about the chores that revolve around them. You drive somewhere to pick up shavings, you drive home and then you have to unload and store them. You strip the stall and add the new shavings. Sometimes you add extra shavings to an already bedded stall. Then you have to keep the stall clean and pick it at least twice per day. What a pain (unless you're not the one doing all the chores). However, you're still spending money on shavings *and* on the labor involved in keeping up the stalls.

If you keep your horses naturally, you'll not only save money but also the time and effort involved in the extra chores. That time and money can be spent elsewhere... like spending more **quality time** with your horse that doesn't involve picking a stall or putting on a blanket.

NATURAL HORSE CARE SAVINGS

Think for a minute how expensive horse blankets are. Many people own a wardrobe of blankets for their horses that cost enough to feed a small country. No wonder horses get the reputation of being expensive.

Human thought patterns, traditional beliefs and great marketing hype are what cause horses to be expensive.

If we keep our horses naturally, many expenses go out the window. We can also use that money to focus on more important things when it comes to our horses, such as their foundation for health.

By kicking your horses out of the stalls and not blanketing, you can save a significant amount of money. Who doesn't want that?

WHEN TO BLANKET YOUR HORSE

Please don't read this and kick your sick or elderly, always-blanketed, unnaturally kept horse out in the cold. One situation I can think of where a horse may need to be blanketed is if a horse is ill. For example, I know a natural hoof care professional who lives in Canada. He emphasizes that even in Canada, with their severe winters, he doesn't blanket his horses unless there's a reason, such as them being sick.

From this point forward, I would suggest learning how to keep a naturally healthy horse so she can stay healthy throughout the winter months without blanketing.

WHAT HORSES DON'T NEED IN COLD WEATHER

➢ A cozy stall bedded with shavings
➢ A heated barn
➢ A blanket
➢ Extra grain (horses DO NOT need grain to stay warm, instead increase forage)
➢ Limited movement

WHAT HORSES DO NEED IN COLD WEATHER

➢ Plenty of free choice grass hay (low in NSC)
➢ Water (at times you may need to warm it for them so they'll drink enough during colder weather)
➢ Plenty of free choice, loose, *unrefined* sea salt
➢ Shelter and wind blocks to get out of the elements, if they choose. Some horses will choose to be out in the snow, rain, etc. It should be up to them to decide.
➢ Allow plenty of movement. Again, movement plays a huge role in a naturally healthy horse, especially in the winter months when they need extra movement to produce body heat and keep their muscles loose.
➢ Additional nutritional support, NOT grain, in a situation where a horse has trouble keeping weight on.

Overall, the horse keeping practice of blanketing your horse is unnecessary and can also be detrimental to your horse's health.

PART III: CREATING A NATURAL HABITAT

Creating an environment for your horse that closely mimics that of wild horses is critical to her health, well-being and soundness. Without this core ingredient, your horse keeping practices will be inferior at best.

This may seem like an impossible task, but in reality, it's a matter of first understanding some basic core principles. In the next few chapters, I'll present to you some strategies that are *outside the norm* that you may want to consider incorporating into your horse keeping practices.

NATURAL HORSE BOARDING AND ENCOURAGING MOVEMENT

"You have to decide to chase after knowledge so passionately that you're constantly looking back thinking about how little you used to know."
~ Nicholas Cardot

THE FIRST RULE

When you think of a domesticated horse, how do you picture it? What does its surroundings look like? The average person may picture a healthy horse in a comfortable stall sticking her head out the door to say hi. The barn she lives in is immaculate and doesn't smell like horses live there. Or, you may picture horses grazing on lush green pastures where they look happy, fat and perfectly content.

Traditional boarding situations that include keeping horses in stalls, small paddocks or grazing on lush green pastures are different than natural boarding. Natural boarding is part of a well-rounded natural horse care program.

The first rule of natural horse care is to implement a natural boarding system.

The biggest difference between wild and domesticated horses is *movement*. Wild horses move about 20 miles per day. Does *your* horse move that much in a day? Movement in both horses and humans is one of the most important ingredients for optimal health.

The less we move, the more our health declines. This same concept holds true, if not *more so*, for our equine companions.

But you say, "I ride my horse every day." Come on, does that come close to 20 miles per day? You may ride your horse for 1-2 hours, several times a week, put her up in a stall or small paddock, and that's it. From there, her food is brought to her twice per day and she barely has to walk to her water. The water trough may be just a few feet away from her feed trough. Wow! What a life. That's not much different than you sitting around most of the time in your recliner chair in front of the TV eating donuts and potato chips, and having your parent or significant other bring you everything you need. You don't even have to go to the grocery store.

In all seriousness, this way of horse keeping is what causes more lameness issues and other health problems. If we were to follow the first rule of natural horse care, we would create a boarding arrangement encouraging our horses to use their natural instincts to stimulate movement, as well as other natural behaviors that are essential to a sound healthy horse.

The second rule of natural horse care is to IMPLEMENT a natural boarding system.

There are plenty of old wives' tales on horse keeping practices that are not in the best interest of your horse. These practices vary and are far from what our horses need naturally. For example, there are all kinds of products and information on the market that will educate you on the different ways you can build a 12 x 12 stall with small runs coming out from the stall area. This sounds more like we're building something for a cave-dwelling animal rather than a horse.

What about the small paddock or "dry lot" solution? Have you ever observed your horse when she is contained in one of these small areas? How much does she move? Her biggest excitement may be you feeding her twice per day. Let's not forget the **chemically fertilized,** treated, weed-free, lush green pasture which is a founder trap. You may think, at least my horse will be allowed to move 24/7. What about the vet bills and possible lameness problems you may end up dealing with?

Maybe these traditional ways of horse keeping work for you and maybe they don't. On that note, here is a startling fact to think about. This statement came from Walt Taylor, co-founder of the American Farrier's Association, and a member of the World Farrier's Association and Working Together for Equines programs:

> *Of the 122 million equines found around the world, no more than 10 percent are clinically sound. Some 10 percent (12.2 million) are clinically, completely and unusably lame. The remaining 80 percent (97.6 million) of these equines are some-what lame... and could not pass a soundness evaluation or test. [American Farrier's Journal, November/2000 v 26,   #6, p. 5]*

When I first saw these numbers, I was amazed. If you look at the date, those facts were presented in *November of 2000*. Do you think it's much better now? I doubt it. We've just scratched the surface of working toward the kind of mind shift needed to turn something like this around. Something to consider is that by wild horse standards, domestic horses are neither healthy nor sound.

WHAT DOES THE FIRST RULE OF NATURAL HORSE CARE HAVE TO DO WITH A HEALTHY HORSE?

The wealth of information gathered through research on wild horses shows that their domesticated counterparts will *thrive* if their environment takes into consideration one of their most basic needs *movement*.

In order for a horse to obtain optimal health, she must be allowed to thrive physically, mentally and emotionally. Through providing a natural boarding system that stimulates movement versus causing less movement, we're one step closer to horses who will *thrive* in domestication with minimal health problems.

Don't let learning more about natural horse care and natural boarding intimidate you, and don't keep doing what you're doing just because you think it's too hard to create a natural environment for your horse. Instead, understand things more from your horse's point of view and learn all you can about implementing a natural boarding system that works for both you *and* your horse.

ENCOURAGE MOVEMENT

Mother Nature intended for horses to move almost constantly. Horses in the wild move up to, if not more than, 20 miles per day. As a result, they can forge a beautiful, naturally shaped hoof, and their bodies are kept in peak condition for the demands placed on them in the wild.

As a horse guardian, it's your responsibility to provide an environment for your horse that closely mimics what Mother Nature intended. Again, we must observe how horses live in the wild and understand that they move up to 20 miles per day; therefore, you must do everything you can to encourage more movement in your horse.

HOW DO YOU ENCOURAGE MORE MOVEMENT?

It's time to lose the stall. If your horse is kept in a small dry lot or paddock then that's better than a stall, but it's still not a good solution. The alternative that most people think is the only other option is a large pasture, but that's not a good solution, either, if the soil is unbalanced and it's heavily fertilized using chemical fertilizers. Another challenge is that not everyone has a large amount of land.

Instead, set up a natural boarding arrangement using a concept called Paddock Paradise. It's a track system for horses and your horse will love it. A Paddock Paradise can be implemented on small or large acreage. The only limitation is your imagination. It's a model for safe, natural horse keeping, hoof care, and the healing and rehabilitation of lame horses.

This natural boarding concept is intended to encourage constant movement, as nature intended, as well as allow horses to behave according to their instincts. As a result, you'll have a healthier horse mentally, physically and emotionally.

Usually, when I introduce this concept to someone they think it's going to be too hard and too expensive to set up. However, it actually *requires little work and expense*, and the track can be set up in an afternoon depending on its size and how elaborate you decide to make it.

The longer you have your track system set up, the more ideas you'll come up with to implement and manage it. It's a brilliant system that I've personally used since April 2006. Remember, the more movement, the healthier your horse.

Something I would like to share, I've never seen a barefoot horse's hooves as pretty as my own horses who are kept on a Paddock Paradise. The reason? They're constantly moving and they forge very different hooves than those I see on customers' horses that I trim who aren't on a Paddock Paradise track system.

It's a simple concept that's easy to implement.

To get started, first read my review of the book *Paddock Paradise - A Guide to Natural Horse Boarding* by Jaime Jackson, and then see if you can fit this concept into your horse keeping practices. You can find a reference to the review in the Online Resources section of this book.

7 WARNING SIGNS THAT YOUR HORSE KEEPING IS INFERIOR

What's the *first* horse keeping practice that benefits the overall health of the horse?

Imagine that you've just walked out to your barn or you've arrived at your boarding facility excited to spend time with your horse. She whinnies for you and as you approach her stall she tries hard to stick her cute nose through the bars to greet you. As you pull her out of the stall, she steps out somewhat stiff, which is not unusual. You don't think anything of it because you're used to it; you may even think it's *normal*.

As equine caregivers, we often wonder if what we're doing for our horses is in their best interest. Is it possible that your horse keeping is *inferior* and your horse is trying to tell you something? What your horse is probably trying to tell you is that you're breaking the first rule of natural horse care.

WHAT'S THE MISSING INGREDIENT

Most equine caregivers would love to optimize their horse keeping practices, but first it's important to be aware of the warning signs that point to inferior horse keeping. Here are seven warning signs that should cause you to rethink your horse keeping strategies. These warning signs are all a side effect of one single ingredient that's missing from most equine horse keeping programs.

Movement

Along with movement comes increased circulation throughout the body. Stalled horses can't move enough to maintain adequate circulation. On top of that, add a horse who's shod and we have further and *significantly* decreased circulation. What does this mean to you?

You have created a horse who:
1) Gets stiff
2) Has poor hoof quality
3) Requires more frequent hoof care = increased hoof care bills
4) Has muscles and ligaments that lose tone
5) Has increased probability of injury
6) Is more prone to illness and increased vet bills
7) Has increased displaced behavior (i.e. cribbing, weaving, aggression, etc.)

THINK THE OPPOSITE OF WHAT YOU THINK IS "NORMAL"

I've come to realize over the years that most of the lessons I teach have a lot to do with a mind shift. That mind shift usually requires you to *think the opposite* of what you think is *normal* by domestic horse standards. So what's the opposite of my seven warning signs list above?

A horse who is allowed to move constantly through the day and night will, by default,

1) Experience minimal or no stiffness (especially in barefoot horses)
2) Have increased hoof quality (in barefoot horses)
3) Require little trimming (in barefoot horses) = decreased hoof care bills
4) Have muscle and ligaments that are toned and well developed
5) Have decreased incidences of injury
6) Be less prone to illness and have minimal vet bills
7) Become a more physically, mentally and emotionally balanced equine companion, free of displaced behaviors

Again, the common denominator of inferior and optimal horse keeping is *movement*.

THE MOST IMPORTANT HORSE KEEPING PRINCIPLES

So, what's all this fuss about movement? If you've gotten this far in the book, you've probably gathered that I harp a lot on the importance of movement. What you'll come to find is that this is the most critical piece of having a horse that truly THRIVES *versus just* SURVIVES. It's the most important piece of the puzzle to having a naturally healthy horse.

If you do nothing else but get this one ingredient right, you'll be about 98% ahead of most horse guardians who think they're doing what's best for their horses.

I often hear the objection that it's illogical to compare our domestic horses to wild horses and, therefore, creating an environment based on that of the wild horse won't work. There's a lot of truth in that, and here's why - they say it will not work for us, and *that*'s the biggest part of our horses' problem. It goes back to this truth...

It may be what's best for every horse, but it's not what's best for every human.

In other words, the human feels it's too hard to implement a natural horse care program when, in reality, the concepts I believe so deeply in and teach to others, simplifies horse keeping and saves money in the long run. And as an added bonus, it produces a naturally healthy horse.

The biggest hurdle I've found is shifting people's way of thinking about their traditional practices. First of all, our horses want to move like nature intended. It's in their DNA. They weren't meant to be kept in small 12 x 12 stalls or small paddocks that cause limited movement. They weren't meant to be fed only 2-3 large meals per day. For us to be selfish and not set up an environment for our horses that closely mimics what Mother Nature intended is not in the best interest of our horses.

THE HORSE KEEPING PRINCIPLES PRIORITY LIST

There is a priority system I use when it comes to keeping my horses naturally. I also teach this system to my clients and recommend that they use this prioritized list in their own horse keeping program.

If these concepts are not used and prioritized in this order, then you're less likely to set up the optimal situation for your horse. Not only that, but if your horse is barefoot, this priority list is even more important because having a barefoot horse will not work, or will be inferior at best, without these three prioritized ingredients. You'll also have little chance of fully rehabilitating a lame horse, if at all.

The List

The list of ingredients that *you must* understand *in this order* is as follows:

1) Movement
2) Diet
3) Hoof Care

This order may be surprising. I'll explain the reasoning behind it. Imagine horses in the wild. They move almost constantly; up to, if not more than, 20 miles per day. As they move, they seek out various plant sources. They don't eat large amounts of lush green grass and they don't eat huge meals at one time; instead, they eat a variety of foodstuffs as they move from location to location. Not only that, those foodstuffs are not artificially processed!

So what happens by default?

> *They move constantly (#1 - movement) in order to obtain food and water (#2 - diet). They forge, <u>through movement</u>, a naturally shaped hoof (#3 - hoof care) for their bodies and for the terrain they live on. Therefore, their hooves function optimally for them. They self trim because they get so much movement.*

Although research of wild horses proves to us that what I just shared with you is true, how can that theory work in domestication?

On several occasions, I've discussed a concept called the Paddock Paradise track system. I believe that until we come up with a better way, this is the best solution for keeping a naturally healthy horse and encouraging more movement - especially for those who don't have the luxury of owning large amounts of land.

MY EXPERIENCES WITH THESE HORSE KEEPING PRINCIPLES

As of July 2011, I have three horses as part of my family. One is 25 years old, another is 22 and one is 5. This is just a small sample of the multitude of horses out there; however, these three horses have taught me a lot about the importance of movement.

The 25 year old is an Appendix Quarter Horse mare (Faith). She's a retired racehorse who's had multiple injuries over her lifetime, and she has many obvious scars as a result. When I got her, she was already in her early teens. Now that I look back, it's amazing she was as sound as she was when she came into my life.

I soon found out that she had multiple problems. She had arthritis, she had problems keeping weight on and she was a "bleeder." A bleeder is a common problem racehorses and many barrel horses have. The first time I saw blood come out of her nose, I immediately thought it was something serious. But I soon learned it could be controlled and managed through her diet. As an added bonus, she came with severe mental and emotional baggage - that was a lot of fun!

The best thing about Faith is how much she loves to move. Despite all the injuries she had through her life, most being to her legs, hips or hoof region, I feel that her movement attribute is what has kept her sound. She's still going strong today at the grand old age of 25, and her arthritis is hardly noticeable anymore. I also don't feed her any kind of joint supplement or processed ingredients.

Many hoof care professionals have problems with horses at this age bringing their hind legs up onto a hoof stand. Although I'm always considerate of a horse's range of motion, meaning in this context how far they can comfortably raise their legs, Faith doesn't have issues with me using the hoof stand when needed. The futurity horses (3-4 year olds) in our area can't hold a candle to her, in my opinion, when it comes to soundness and overall health. I believe that has a lot to say for the naturally healthy horse concept.

Horse breeds such as Thoroughbreds and Arabians are probably the easiest to take barefoot as long as you allow them to get plenty of movement. These two breeds love to move. They will forge the most beautiful, naturally shaped hoof you'll ever see. It's all about the number one ingredient... *movement*.

Now for a little information on my 22 year-old gelding (Dillon). He's the one who forced me to learn about natural hoof care. I wasn't always a barefoot advocate. I used to love the sound of a shod horse walking down a concrete alleyway. Wow, things are different now. Now when I hear that sound, I first look at the horse's hooves and read the hoof. I can't help but think about the amount of shock going through that horse's body by walking on the concrete with metal shoes. I also think about the poor circulation and her imbalances, both hoof and body.

I empathize with that horse having to compensate for all those things *and* carry the weight of both saddle and rider. Additionally, the saddle is usually ill fitting, the rider is mediocre at best, and there's little or no communication between the two resulting in force rather and understanding and partnership.

It's amazing how forgiving horses are and what they do to compensate for our inadequacies. That will always blow my mind!

Okay, back to Dillon. Dillon came into my life in his mid teens. Now that I look back, he had what's called a forward foot syndrome and was very "flat footed," which basically means the internal structures of his hoof dropped down to an unnatural and unhealthy position in his hoof capsule.

I had all kinds of problems with him staying sound. During that time of trying to help Dillon, what do you think I focused on? The hoof. I now know that's a *stupid thing* to do. Not only is it stupid, it can cause more problems when that's all you focus on.

After a lot of expensive, fancy shoeing and no results, I started looking for an alternative. Looking for an alternative was easy for me to do because I was already all about alternative approaches to my own health, as well as the care of my dogs and cats.

Once I started to research and look for answers, it was history after that, but needless to say, Dillon has been a tough case. The good thing is that I believe he's healthier now at the age of 22 than he was when he came to me in his early teens. At least I'm on the right track. Anytime I wasn't on the right track, Dillon let me know.

He's sound, his weight is good and he's still rideable. The lameness issue was not the only thing I had to address with Dillon. The problems that caused the lameness were many. It wasn't just about pulling the shoes and doing a natural trim. It was about addressing underlying issues.

He's a big horse who loves to eat. He's prone to laminitis and I had to overcome a few cases with him. But now he's a much different horse.

The key ingredient to him becoming sound and healthy is the amount of movement he gets on the track system.

He also has a playmate in my younger horse. Neither of my older horses look nor act their age, which is an excellent example of the naturally healthy horse concept at work, resulting in quality of life and longevity.

During the time that I was going through all of that with Dillon, I wasn't as fortunate as most of you who are reading this today. At that time, there wasn't nearly the amount of information and research available on natural hoof care. Nor were there as many competent hoof care professionals around to help.

A lot has changed in the last 10 years. Although people are more aware of the barefoot movement now, another problem has surfaced. People may take their horses barefoot, but they're *still* only focusing on the hoof.

Natural hoof care will not work if the entire package is not taken into consideration. Without first addressing the overall health and well-being of your horse, and the underlying cause of lameness, you will have on-going problems. This is one reason why people say bare-foot doesn't work.

If you want to keep your horse barefoot and have her stay sound, you have to adopt a natural horse care lifestyle.

As you read this, you may be wondering, "What about your young horse, Ransom?" Well, I haven't forgotten about him. Ransom is very special and he's been a fantastic case study. He's the true test, in my world, of utilizing the naturally healthy horse concept.

Ransom came into my life when he was a year old. As of the writing of this book, he's 5 years of age and he has lived on the track system his entire life (except for his first year). The hooves he has forged through movement are beautiful and functional.

He's never been shod and he's had lots and lots of movement over the four years he's been with me. I started him myself under saddle when he was almost 3 and I haven't asked much of him, just yet. Like I said, he's *almost* fully developed physically.

I don't want to interfere with his growth. However, I have been developing both his mind and body without the weight of saddle or rider. *I don't have to ride him to develop him and our relationship.*

The kind of horse development he has received far outweighs the vast number of "professionally trained" young horses within a hundred mile radius. Not only that, he's much healthier and more sound. He's changed drastically in his physical makeup between 3 and 5 years of age.

My goal for Ransom, as it is for all horses, is quality of life and longevity.

I expect him to still be sound and rideable well into his thirties. Is it possible? Yes it is

Longevity in a horse is usually a non-existent goal for many in the horse industry because most think of horses as disposable objects. They're usually broken down and lame by the time they're 4 or 5 years of age. If they're *lucky* enough to make it into their twenties, they usually pass away in their *early* twenties carrying with them emotional trauma, baggage and physical pain.

The three principles I shared with you, **movement**, **diet** and **hoof care**, are only the tip of the iceberg when it comes to keeping a naturally healthy horse. The concepts are actually simple; however, the amount of information on this subject can feel somewhat overwhelming.

If you stick around *Soulful Equine*, we intend to eliminate that which is overwhelming and help you dive into each of these areas, as well as various other subjects on natural horse care. We'll look in-depth on specific subjects through our online courses, interactive learning environments and various educational materials.

ENCOURAGE SOCIALIZATION

A natural boarding arrangement would not be complete without the subject of equine socialization. Mother Nature intended horses to live in a herd and have interaction with other horses. In the wild, horses depend heavily on their unique social units called bands, which are just family or extended family. Their highly structured society demonstrates their need for interaction as they play, compete for dominance and rest in the sun.

Allowing your horse to live and interact with a herd or a companion is important to her overall health and well-being.

You may be afraid to allow your horse to socialize and you may not realize this is a fundamental need for her. You may say to me, "But

I'm afraid my horse will get hurt if I put her with another horse." This *could* happen, but most likely, if your horse is properly introduced to a herd, the initial process of becoming part of it is less stressful on everyone, including your horse. It's more detrimental to your horse's mental and physical well-being if you don't allow her to live with another companion or other herd members. She's likely to develop displaced behaviors such as cribbing, weaving, aggression, etc.

From an athletic standpoint, it can also provide additional exercise since horses like to move as a herd. A companion or other herd mates will help encourage more movement, which will result in a more naturally healthy horse.

If you only have one horse, I would recommend either purchasing another horse or providing some kind of companion for her such as a goat, sheep or cow. The adoption or rescue of an older horse is also an option.

Horses are not meant to be alone!

Having other animals around can help fulfill her basic need for socialization.

SOME NITTY GRITTY TRACK SYSTEM CONCEPTS

Every revolutionary idea seems to evoke three stages of reaction – "1) It's completely impossible – don't waste my time, 2) It's possible but it's not worth doing, 3) I said it was a good idea all along." ~ Arthur C. Clarke

THE SCOOP ON HORSE POOP

Many years ago, Sharon (Co-founder of Soulful Equine) and I decided to drive to Glen Rose, Texas, to visit the Fossil Rim Wildlife Center. As it states on their website, *The Fossil Rim Wildlife Center* exists to aid in the conservation of animal species under the threat of extinction in the wild." The experience was fascinating, and if you're ever in Texas it's a great place to visit. It's also an organization you can put on your list for donations each year.

WHITE RHINOCEROS AND THE MANURE PILE

We took a tour of the grounds in our car. Along the way we saw giraffes and other wonderful animals. The giraffes liked to stick their whole head through your car window to say hi. All I could think of was that their cute little noses and mouths reminded me of my horses'.

As we came to the end of the tour, we stopped to watch a white rhinoceros with her baby at her side. Our attention was more on the baby than the mother because she was so cute. I had never seen a real live rhinoceros baby before. We stayed parked, watching and observing them.

I noticed that in the middle of the area they lived in, there was a huge dung/manure pile. The pile was probably about 8-10 feet wide and maybe at least 5 feet tall. All of a sudden, the mother rhinoceros walked right over to the pile of manure, turned around, backed right up to the edge of it and pooped! I couldn't believe my eyes. I thought, "How cool is that!" The thought immediately entered my mind that if only I could teach my horses to do the same thing that would be wonderful. Manure management would be a breeze.

STUD PILES AND HORSE BEHAVIOR

Witnessing the rhinoceros and her large poop pile caused me to open my eyes to the importance of learning more about equine behavior patterns. Before that day I didn't think much about *teaching* my horses to manage their own manure. Little did I realize, they do it naturally if I would pay attention. Maybe I could even add a little guidance and direct the poop placement.

Since April 2006, I've kept my horses on a track boarding system that encourages them to move constantly, similar to how they would in the wild. It's a powerful natural boarding concept. The concept is discussed more in a book by Jaime Jackson called *Paddock Paradise: A Guide to Natural Horse Boarding*. You can find a reference to a review of the book I wrote in the Online Resources section.

Without going into the details of horse behavior, I'm going to keep it simple for you. There's a significant amount of wild horse research that addresses the subject of territorial marking known as *stud piles* also called *dung piles*. Don't allow the term "stud piles" to confuse you and cause you to think that it *only* applies to stallions, because it doesn't. It mostly has to do with relative dominance or the pecking order in a herd of horses, be it wild or domesticated.

Those who search for bands of wild horses know that stud piles are the first sign of horse activity. These large piles of manure are simply territorial markings. This form of scent marking causes *repeated dunging* in the same place. Hmm... how can we use the horse's natural behavior, the concept of stud piles and repeated dunging to our advantage?

HORSE TERRITORIAL MARKINGS AND MANURE CONTROL

In Jaime Jackson's book about the paddock paradise, he discusses stud piles and suggests that in order to keep more in line with a wild horse model, we should deliberately leave a certain amount of manure within the track. He says there are two reasons for this, *dominance* and *copraphagous* behaviors.

After witnessing the rhinoceros many years prior, along with observation and researching wild horse behavior, this made total sense to me. It was logical and I wanted to do everything I could not to deprive my domesticated partners of any opportunity to use their natural instinctive behaviors.

On the track, I started to form stud piles. At first, I allowed my horses to choose where they wanted to create the piles. I then came along each day, cleaned up the manure and placed it into a pile along the side of the track where they had marked. Over the first week or two, I helped my horses form about four or five stud piles. Stud piles can be several feet wide and as high as 2 or 3 feet. The piles I formed on the track usually were not more than 1 or 2 feet high.

What I noticed over time was that by simply creating stud piles, it caused my horses to poop in the same places on a consistent basis. The simple concept is that your horses will actually start to create the stud piles for you and then you take it from there.

Important lessons I learned when managing stud piles on the track.

- ➤ It's important to manage the piles daily, if possible, or the radius of the poop relative to the stud pile will gradually increase, which is something we want to avoid. I have three horses and I walk the quarter mile track once per day to scoop poop and put out hay. It usually takes me about 15 minutes in total.
- ➤ Ideally, remove manure piles weekly or every other week. One way to manage the amount of manure on the track is to remove the piles, but only after your horses have established their stud pile locations. I've found that once established they'll continue to return to that same place to poop.
- ➤ Don't mess it up by getting lazy. As long as you continue to manage the piles, your horses will use them. Countless times, I've witnessed my own horses deliberately walking to a stud pile and pooping directly on top of the pile. This stuff works!
- ➤ Do not throw manure over the fence wherever you want to discourage stud pile creation. The horse will sense that the manure is still there and continue to poop in that same place.

OTHER HORSE MANURE MANAGEMENT STRATEGIES

If you find that your horse attempts to create a stud pile in a place you don't want him to, get on top of the situation and remove the manure as soon as you can. It's best not to allow build up or your horse will continue to poop in that location. I'll usually remove the manure and place it on the nearest stud pile.

Do not feed your horses next to or near the stud piles. Keep hay away from the piles for health reasons, but also to discourage your horses from pooping in their hay. I personally feed on the ground and provide various mixes of hay around the track to encourage movement.

I have three versions of the track system. The track system I set up loops around about 6 acres. I have a smaller track system with footing that helps with keeping that area somewhat dried up during the wetter times of the year. The stud pile concept works in this smaller area as well.

See our Online Resources section for a picture of an area next to my mega stud pile (compost pile) that is outside the horse pen. Even though the pile is on the other side of the fence, the horses choose to poop right next to the large pile. I pick up this poop every morning, but as you will see in the pictures, my three horses choose to poop in that area. It makes it much easier to manage manure.

The concept of stud piles and horses pooping in one location is nothing new. However, if we understand more about horses' natural behavior and their tendencies, we can work with them versus against them. This can also result in less work for us as well.

HOW TO USE HORSE WATERING BEHAVIOR FOR POWERFUL NATURAL BOARDING

In the section of this book called *The Scoop on Horse Poop*, I discussed the importance of manure when it comes to relative dominance in a herd, and how you can utilize a horse's natural behaviors to your advantage for managing manure. This section continues to provide information on bridging that gap between the world of the wild horse and the domestic horse.

Closely mimicking a more natural environment for our horses, by default, can result in a healthy equine partner that will live a long quality life. As an added bonus, we may even see a decrease in our veterinarian bills.

MY ACCIDENTAL HORSE WATERING HOLE

Each year I usually have someone do dirt work on my horse track system to smooth over any huge ruts or holes my horses created in areas where they love to lay down. Sometimes I bring in more pea gravel or sand and put it on the track or around the barn. One sandy area on the track that is close to the barn developed a *huge* crater in the ground over time. Initially, I decided to cover it up and smooth it over until we ended up getting a significant amount of rainfall over a six-month period. Every time it rained, that big hole in the ground filled up with water.

I started to notice a pattern develop in my small herd. Each time after a rainfall, they would mosey on over to the water hole, drink water, paw, and sometimes roll in the watering hole. This of course made the hole bigger.

What was interesting is that they went out of their way to drink the water out of the water hole rather than drinking out of the water trough. Even though I filter my horses' water and keep their troughs clean, they chose to drink rainwater at ground level from the water-ing hole. At first, interesting, but then, not so much since that's what horses do in the wild.

Since creating my track system, I always wanted a watering hole for my horses. Well, be careful what you wish for... mine appeared over time. Needless to say, I decided to keep it.

HORSE WATERING HOLE BEHAVIOR

The horses love it! During the hot summer months here in Texas, I keep it filled up with water. It's fun to watch their behavior around the watering hole and it can be quite fascinating at times. What I have noticed about my own horses is that they love taking mud baths and pawing in the watering hole. Another thing I've noticed is that they like to soak their hooves in the water. That helps with providing some moisture to their hooves, if needed.

Even though excessive moisture is not good for natural hoof form, a watering hole where the horse may not stay for long, will contribute to their overall health and well-being. Plus, have you ever heard of how beneficial mud baths are?

I believe horses understand the benefits of mud more than we do.

There are times one of my horses may take a mud bath and then head over to a nearby sandy area to roll and dry off. Something to consider is that these watering hole behaviors can help with your horse's coat conditioning as well as protection from insects. I notice they prefer to cake on the mud during the times of year when insects are at their worst. I tend to save money on fly spray when they do this.

I know what you're thinking. You don't want your beautiful clean horse to be caked in mud that you have to clean off. First of all, horses aren't meant to be sparkling clean all the time. If it was up to them they'd prefer to be dirty. Have you ever noticed horses love to roll right after you clean them up? Just remember, all you have to do is wait until the next day and most of the mud is gone from their coats.

WHAT ABOUT THE WATER TROUGH?

My horses still drink out of their water troughs even though they now have a watering hole. A horse will determine its own daily watering schedule. Sometimes they may use the water trough and other times the watering hole. That being said,

I strategically place the water troughs on the track to encourage more natural movement.

An interesting behavior my horses will exhibit on the track is during their camping time. Camping is when horses will come together and stand around looking like zombies. In all seriousness, they rest for short periods of time, dozing on occasion, usually while standing.

They love camping under a shed I have on the track that also has a water trough. I've noticed that they choose that particular shed *when* I keep the water trough there. They usually gather and stand right around that trough taking turns drinking like they're in a spa area. I've experimented with moving the trough to different locations under the shed and they exhibit the same behavior - they'll stand right around the trough and sometimes directly over it.

Learning more about horse watering hole behaviors can help you continue to improve your natural boarding arrangement. Sometimes, as in my case, a small watering hole that the horse can drink, bathe and take a mud bath in is all that is needed. If you're like me and you're not one of the fortunate ones who have a nice pond on your property, you may need to get a little creative. I like to keep things simple, so try not to over analyze this concept.

The important thing is that I listened to and observed my horses in order to understand their needs.

Through observation, and allowing the watering hole to remain, I was able to more closely mimic a wild horse environment for my domesticated partners. The fun part is that my horses, with a little help from Mother Nature, created it. Maybe you'll get that lucky too.

PART IV: FOUNDATIONAL NUTRITION

Putting a good foundational nutrition program in place for your horse, and for you, can optimize the ability to stay healthy. Consistently incorporating foundational nutrition into your horse program can help prevent disease. This section introduces you to this concept and arms you with information for making more informed choices when it comes to your horse's diet.

AN INTRODUCTION TO EQUINE DIET CONSIDERATIONS

"When diet is wrong medicine is of no use. When diet is correct medicine is of no need."
~ Ancient Ayurvedic Proverb

A CONSISTENTLY HEALTHY HORSE

Have you ever wondered if you're providing your horse with a good base of foundational nutrition? What is foundational nutrition? That's a somewhat loaded question that results in a variety of answers depending on whom you talk with. Throughout this chapter, I'll explain my view on foundational nutrition, what it includes, and how it relates to your horse so she can *consistently* stay healthy.

A steady pattern I've noticed throughout my adult life is that the majority of people have difficulty staying healthy themselves, so I question how they can possibly understand what's healthy for their horses. For example, I once took a course from a well-known instructor who included information on equine nutrition in the course material. During breaks, that same instructor would walk outside and smoke a cigarette. After seeing that, it caused me to question the credibility of this person as it pertained to educating others about horse health.

I'm a firm believer in setting good examples. To me, it's not much different than an overweight doctor trying to educate me on how to eat right. What I've found is that those who don't take their own health seriously, frequently struggle to understand the best approach to take when it comes to the health of their equine companions. Additionally, they're often easily swayed by popular opinion.

Some people may argue that good human health practices have nothing to do with horses; however, there are many similarities, not to mention some basic fundamentals that must be in place in the diet for both horses and humans.

THE CONCEPT OF FOUNDATIONAL NUTRITION

Before I go much further, I'd like to introduce to you a concept called foundational nutrition.

"Foundational nutrition is the combination of nutrients your horse needs on a regular basis so she can consistently stay free from disease and health issues." ~ Stephanie Krahl

One step up from foundational nutrition is something called therapeutic nutrition.

What I've found is that the key to a horse staying consistently healthy is to educate people and help them understand that there's a foundational level of health that a horse must obtain. By providing a good foundation on a regular basis, therapeutic nutrition is usually no longer needed. Once equine guardians understand this, they'll usually continue to keep a good foundational program in place.

When a problem arises with a horse that's health related, the first thing that's usually addressed are symptoms rather than the underlying cause(s). Sometimes even holistic health care practitioners jump right to the therapeutic side of the equation instead of addressing the foundation first. Again, make sure you have a good foundational base to build on.

SO WHERE DO YOU START?

A frequent problem in the equine industry today is that the majority of guardians have holes in their foundational program and this is where most problems originate. With so much conflicting information on equine nutrition, you may ask yourself, "Where do I start?" By taking the concept that **nutrition comes from food**, you have to first start by looking at your horse's lifestyle. Where are the deficiencies coming from?

If you want to start adding nutrition into your horse's life, you have to first start looking at what **your horse's lifestyle is like.** So, the first question you have to ask yourself before wasting a lot of money on feeding supplements or expensive commercial feeds is, "Does my horse need them?" *Does she REALLY need them?*

Is there a need for *basic* supplementation on a consistent basis in the world today? Keep in mind that I'm talking about basic foundational nutrition, not therapeutic nutrition. Where do you start?

> *If your horse has any kind of symptom, foundational nutrition is where you start.*

Beyond that, whatever diagnostic procedures you use, whether it's blood testing, hair analysis or muscle testing, you then add therapeutic nutrition on top of the foundation. But always keep in mind that it's important to first start with foundational nutrition.

NATURE'S FOUNDATION FOR HEALTH AND HOW IT RELATES TO YOUR HORSE

Nutrition is a huge subject that's both a science and an art. Keeping that in mind, it's not realistic to cover it in great detail in a short course or presentation. I can cover this in more depth, but due to the scope of this book, what I will cover are some basic elements you need to consider when it comes to keeping your horse naturally.

> *I believe diet is one of the most important ingredients to overcoming health problems in our horses as well as in ourselves.*

As I mentioned in the previous section, I've found that the key to a horse staying consistently healthy is for her to first obtain a solid *foundational level* of health. This is an important concept to grasp.

By providing good foundational nutrition on a regular basis, common health problems are usually decreased and they can even become non-existent. Most horses are not on a good, consistent foundational program. Over time, this can cause various symptoms or problems to arise.

When I talk about foundational nutrition, most people think it's just about giving your horse hay, the most popular processed feed on the market, and a mix of supplements that don't provide optimally bioavailable forms of minerals. This is far from the truth.

What is fed to horses today is **highly processed** and not in-line with what their bodies need to stay healthy. Most people feed their horse like they feed themselves, utilizing highly processed foodstuffs that contain little or no nutritional value.

NATURE'S FOUNDATION FOR HEALTH

The importance of nature's foundation for health is something that's usually overlooked by most equine guardians. If a horse's body does not get the nutrients it needs from food, the body cannot function and health declines. Eventually, symptoms will worsen and your horse may die prematurely.

A return to health must begin with a change of diet.

You must feed your horses more fresh and raw, non-processed (or minimally processed) whole foods. Additionally, you need to supplement your horse's diet in order to replace what is missing and to pay back the nutritional debts created by years of poor diet.

When I say supplement, you must be careful because just like food, **supplements can also be highly processed**, resulting in the loss of the natural co-factors necessary for the body to utilize them. The nutrients you feed to your horse must be in an optimally bioavailable form.

To ensure that your horses, as well as you and your family, are getting all of the necessary nutrients, you must first provide nature's foundation for health:

➢ Enzymes - naturally found in raw food but destroyed by heat (processing). They help the body digest food, so the nutrients can be fully utilized. Enzymes are completely destroyed in most processed feeds, especially pelleted feeds. It takes very high temperatures to create a pellet.

➢ Probiotics - beneficial bacteria that naturally strengthen the immune system and produce countless beneficial nutrients. Not all probiotic products for horses are created equal. Probiotics are fragile and can also be destroyed in processing, such as high heat used to create pelleted products.

➢ Whole-Food Vitamins and Minerals – can be made by using nutrient dense, whole, raw foods, and removing only the water and fiber, retaining all the natural co-factors and synergistic micro-nutrients. Provide minerals that are organically chelated and mined directly from natural deposits. Most of what is fed to horses is highly processed and the benefits of whole-food vitamins and minerals are destroyed.

➢ Antioxidants - protective molecules that prevent free radical damage to tissues. They are most abundant in brightly colored whole foods, certain trace minerals and botanicals.

➢ Essential Fatty Acids - these are the good fats that are required for every cell and organ in the body. They help reduce inflammation, inhibit cancer development, improve brain function, regulate organs and glands and protect blood vessels. The body cannot make them, so a direct food source is essential. These good fats are fragile and can immediately start to become rancid if exposed to heat, air or light.

➢ Unrefined Sea Salt - this is salt that has not been refined or processed. Avoid regular table salt, because it has been treated with chemicals such as sulfuric acid or chlorine in order to remove the minerals (which are then sold for other uses). These minerals are referred to as "impurities" in table salt, which is entirely untrue.

Nature's foundation for health is important when it comes to our horses. The nutrients in unprocessed foods work synergistically to provide the body the tools it needs to maintain optimal health.

Keep in mind, as I said above, that supplements and other products you buy for your horse can be **heavily processed**, which cancels out any nutritional value.

By understanding this fundamental concept, and learning how to properly read labels, you'll be able to intelligently select nutrients to include in your horse's diet. This will help her to thrive.

FEEDING COMMERCIAL HORSE FEEDS – WHAT TO CONSIDER

My intent is not to bash particular name brand feeds or give you complete solutions, but rather to provide information to create awareness about the harmful effects of commercial feeds.

If you haven't been concerned about how many horse feed recalls there have been in the last decade, it may be time to think about it and choose your feed wisely. By wisely, I mean not just from a nutritional standpoint but also from a safety standpoint. For example, there have been many articles published over the years by the *Horse Journal* about feed recalls. It's important to be aware and careful because those conveniently, well-packaged and well-marketed horse feeds may not be what is best for your equine companion.

One informative article from the June 2009 Horse Journal was titled, *Grain Quality And Your Horse's Feed.* For those who haven't read it, once you do, you may think twice before making that trip to the feed store.

My intent with this information is to get you to:

1) Think more about what you feed your horse
2) Question all brands; don't trust/assume they're safe for your horse
3) Use a "Back To Basics" approach

Let's face it, it doesn't matter what the subject is, there will be differing opinions - especially when it comes to feeding our equine partners. I've noticed over many years that even people who are considered "experts" on certain subjects in the horse industry don't agree with each other.

There are also times when most people get so bogged down in research that they forget to bring Mother Nature, common sense and intuition into the equation; however, the logical mind wants proof.

What's even more interesting is that most studies contradict each other or come to no logical conclusion, so it comes back to this: who do you believe? I'm not going to tell you *who* to believe. However, I will share with you what I've learned from my experiences and the horses in my care. I will also share what I've learned from some of the *so-called* experts on certain subjects. I have yet to agree completely with any *one* approach.

Since I've been a nutrition fanatic for most of my adult life, it has come in handy when trying to understand what my horses need in their diets. Before I go much further, you're probably wondering whether or not I think every commercial feed is bad.

The answer is no, but I have yet to find one I would feel comfortable feeding or recommending. There are some organic feeds on the market that may be good, but I've only looked at a few and based on the ingredients, still decided not to use them.

ARE YOU LOOKING FOR A MAGIC BULLET OR QUICK FIX?

I fully understand that most people want convenience and that's what we *think* commercial feeds provide us when, in reality, about 99.99% of them are not what's best for your horse. Almost every commercial feed is *heavily processed* and contains ingredients I would never feed to my own horse.

Horse guardians have been brainwashed over the years to believe that horses need grain. What they need is forage, minerals and salt, as well as a variety of whole foods and herbs.

Over the course of many years I've noticed commercial feeds for horses mirroring the *fad diets* that have come along in humans (i.e. low carbohydrate diets, high protein diets, etc.).

Now, due to the epidemic of insulin resistance (IR) in horses, the latest trend is the mass manufacturing of low carbohydrate feeds and supplements. These manufacturers all claim that their products control IR in horses, but it's mostly brilliant marketing and high prices. Who suffers? Our horses. I don't believe the hype.

There is no magic bullet that works as a complete wholistic approach! In addition, there's no such thing as a "complete feed."

The key is to research and gather information in order to make informed decisions.

Remember to tread carefully when listening to experts and be your horse's advocate.

ARE YOU A LITTLE CONFUSED?

I fully understand how difficult it is to grasp concepts that are the opposite of what you've been taught to believe for many years. My intent in this section is to plant a seed, since the complexity on the subject of nutrition is somewhat involved and overwhelming.
What I'll offer you are a few notes to consider:

> ➤ Avoid pelleted feeds of any kind.
> ➤ Avoid pelleted supplements of any kind.
> ➤ Pelleted products are *highly* processed using excessive heat which destroys most of the nutritional value. Are you sure you're getting the best value and is the convenience worth compromising your horse's health?
> ➤ Processed feeds will mold or spoil more quickly than a natural, whole-food grain.
> ➤ Most vitamins in feed mixes aren't stable for very long.
> ➤ Chelated minerals that are used in most feeds may be a waste of money.
> ➤ It's difficult to determine the quality of grains that have been processed or heated. With whole grains, you can check the

color, size, and cleanliness easily.

➢ Do you remember all the pet food recalls? What about all the FDA feed recalls in the last decade?

I could keep going on with this list, but I hope I've given you enough information so you'll give the subject of feeding commercial feeds some thought. I'm sure you've come to the conclusion that I don't feed commercially prepared feeds to my horses. It would take some hard convincing for me to ever do that again.

Let's talk briefly about the *Back to Basics* I mentioned in my opening paragraphs.

BACK TO BASICS

In short, a naturally fed horse means providing whole grains (if needed), plenty of forage, quality salt and minerals instead of heavily processed feeds. Think "whole food form" instead of processed.

I liken it to choosing an apple over a Twinkie or doughnut. Which choice is more likely to provide you the nutrition your body needs for quality of life and longevity?

Usually, the less something is processed and the fewer ingredients it contains, the better the choice.

Remember, minimal or no processing is ideal.

Horse nutrition for the *domesticated horse* is an art *and* a science. Although this needs a significant amount of research, if we stick to what we believe horses would seek out on their own in the wild, then our horses will be better off. This is another example of common sense trumping empirical evidence.

PART V: PREPARATION FOR BAREFOOT

Throughout this book I continue to stress the importance of under-standing the foundational concepts for keeping a naturally healthy horse. In this part, I present core principles about this mystical thing in the horse world called *barefoot*, and I will arm you with plenty of information to get you started.

NATURAL HOOF CARE: A GUIDE TO GETTING STARTED

"A horse that is sound only in shoes is not a sound horse." ~ Steve Dick

AN INTRODUCTION

For at least a decade, I've observed an incredible movement evolving referred to as *natural hoof care*. What's interesting is that most people, like me, started down the road to natural hoof care because of a particular situation. They were either unable to make progress using traditional approaches, or their vet and farrier were at a loss. Other individuals think it might help enhance their horse's perform-ance and health.

Each person and horse situation is different.

One common pattern I've noticed is that usually most people won't consider natural hoof care until they're at a crossroads. Most likely, they've been observing someone else who's setting a good example and/or they've heard about it through the grapevine and want to know more.

A good lesson I learned early on is that it's important not to try to sell someone on taking their horse barefoot or to offer information unless they ask. It's never a good idea to be pushy about anything but rather to set good examples. People usually come around when they see the results and the benefits.

When you love horses as much as I do, this advice is hard to put into practice because the horse is the one that ends up suffering.

In order to help the horse we must first educate the human.

One of the biggest lessons you'll learn when switching from traditional hoof care to natural hoof care is that the hooves are just a small piece of a much bigger picture. Although a horse's hooves are an important piece of the equation, they're usually a symptom and not the underlying cause of lameness. This is where most people think it's just too hard to go barefoot when, in reality, it can simplify things.

Again, what's important? Education and change in thought patterns.

In my case, my then 14-year-old quarter horse gelding, Dillon, caused me to take a look at natural hoof care. He had been in shoes all his life and became increasingly lame even when shod. During that time, I decided to dig for answers.

I then came across Jaime Jackson's book on natural hoof care. After extensive research, I made the decision to pull Dillon's shoes for good and never look back. I'd like to point out that this was during a time when the natural hoof care movement was not as well-known as it is today and there were very few natural hoof care professionals available.

It's also important to note that I had a *slight advantage* because I had learned many aspects of how to trim horses as a teenager. Therefore, I was familiar with the physical ability and coordination it took for using the tools and being under a horse.

If you're starting out today, you'll want to seek out a competent natural hoof care professional to help you. Remember that every situation and horse is different, so it's best *not* to pull your horse's shoes if you have little to no knowledge of how to properly transition her.

After I made the decision to pull Dillon's shoes, my farrier at the time was closed-minded to the idea. As a result, he didn't show up for my next scheduled appointment and dropped me as a customer altogether - simply because I wanted to pull my horse's shoes.

He left me without any help and I knew I would get the same kind of resistance from other traditional farriers in the area. Be prepared for this type of response. It's *still* quite common.

Since the barefoot movement was in its early stages, it was foreign to most people. If they had heard of it, they probably thought it was for crazy people. Based on what I know now, my experience with how my farrier reacted was not uncommon.

That particular farrier handled the situation in an unprofessional manner, and it was clear to me that he did not have my horse's best interests in mind.

From the farrier's perspective, it was not about health and healing but about time and money.

I then arranged for another farrier to pull the shoes on both my horses and then do a flat pasture trim. My plan was to have him pull the shoes and then I would take over from there.

If I were in that same situation today, I'd approach it differently.

I would contact a qualified natural hoof care professional so she could get me started. Also, I would not allow a traditional farrier to trim my horse or pull the shoes, because they could easily cause more harm to a horse, making a bad situation worse.

This can happen if the farrier bruises the sole when carelessly removing the shoe and/or takes material from the bottom of the hoof that may need to stay for protection during the initial transition.

Consequently, the guardian sees her horse tender-footed and in pain and thinks she can't go barefoot, resulting in the horse eventually being re-shod. Unfortunately this comes about due to not understanding how to properly transition a horse and not from an inability to go barefoot.

Any horse can go barefoot.

During the situation with Dillon, I decided that if I wanted things to change, I would have to take matters into my own hands. However, I didn't do it without seeking more knowledge and I didn't make that decision lightly.

I wasn't too worried about my trimming abilities. When I was young, a family friend, who was a farrier, showed me how to do a basic trim and how to properly get under a horse. At least I was a little ahead of things in that area.

I soon found out that those skills, along with my athletic abilities, came in handy when getting under a horse.

When I had the farrier out to pull Dillon's shoes, he commented on what a "flat-footed" horse he was. I'll never forget what he said to me, and it's still just as crystal clear today,

"Once a flat-footed horse, always a flat-footed horse."

Based on what I'd already researched, I knew differently. If only he could see Dillon today. He wouldn't believe it was the same horse. He was the last traditional farrier to ever lay a hand on my horses, and now I do all my own trimming. As of the writing of this book, that was almost ten years ago.

A note on the term "research" - some barefoot experts publicly downgrade those who use the term research when not done by an actual scientist, but research is merely "the collecting of information about a particular subject."

It's unfortunate that our horses suffer while we do formal studies, that often take years, on subjects that are self-evident. Why arrogantly waste time on these studies when mere observation and comparison will work and will change lives, especially when time is of the essence?

Dillon was in bad shape when we first started out, but between my love for Dillon, my passion for learning and the chance to give him a better quality of life, he's now healthy, sound and still rideable. Although Dillon is well into his twenties, he keeps my younger horse in line and gives him a run for his money.

I'm not going to say it was an easy road, because it wasn't. There was a lot of learning involved, but fortunately for all my horses and for me, it was one of the best decisions I ever made.

My statements above are not to imply that all traditional farriers are bad. That's not true. I think in general, they're just trying to make a living and they're doing what they were taught. On the other hand, natural hoof care is a different ball game altogether. I've been applying the principles for a decade, and as natural hoof care evolves, it just keeps getting better.

LOSE THE METAL SHOES

Although I'm all about keeping horses barefoot, there are some situations where this may not be the best choice. Are you surprised?

What I mean by that statement is that barefoot is best for every horse, but it's not necessarily best for every human.

When you decide to pull the shoes on your horse, it's not just about "pulling the shoes" and going barefoot.

There are many other factors involved. It's also not *only about the trim*.

Generally, many people jump on the "barefoot horse bandwagon" for one of two reasons:

1) They're desperate, their horse is completely lame and their vet and farrier are all out of ideas.

2) They think it will increase their horse's competitive edge.

These are not the only reasons you may decide to pull your horse's shoes, but they're the *most* common. Number one above is actually the most common.

So what happens when someone decides to pull their horse's shoes and go against traditional methods of hoof care?

If you're misinformed, if you don't work with a competent natural hoof care professional, and you choose not to educate yourself, then more than likely barefoot will not work in your particular situation.

It may be what's best for your horse, but if you want to continue to be in the dark about understanding what it takes for natural hoof care to work, then pulling your horse's shoes is not right for you.

If you do decide to go the barefoot route, you will be forced to learn about natural horse keeping practices, which is what we educate people about at Soulful Equine. However, when someone hears the words *natural horse care* they usually don't think about *natural hoof care*.

In reality, a naturally healthy horse will also be barefoot.

What it boils down to is that barefoot will not work for you if you only focus on the hoof care side of the equation. It will work if you focus on both hoof care and keeping a naturally healthy horse.

It's not only about pulling the shoes. It must encompass all the concepts of keeping a naturally healthy horse. Horse health and hoof health go hand-in-hand. One will not work without the other.

CORE PRINCIPLES OF NATURAL HOOF CARE

It's important to understand that those who say natural hoof care doesn't work most likely didn't apply all the necessary principles correctly, or at all.

So, What Will Allow Barefoot to Work for Your Horse?

There are three core principles that will allow natural hoof care to work for your horse. You must also understand the order of importance, which is as follows:

1) Movement
2) Diet
3) Hoof Care/The Trim

In order to keep a naturally healthy and sound horse, you must understand that each one of these areas branches off into more detailed information. Being aware of these principles and their importance will put you ahead of others who are struggling with the idea of keeping their horse barefoot.

1) Movement

Lots of movement - this doesn't mean only one or two hours per day of riding or a few hours of turnout. Wild horses move up to 20 miles a day. There are methods that can be applied using a horse's natural tendencies to cause more movement. Movement does not mean out during the day and then in a stall at night. It means 24/7 turnout with equine companionship.

2) Diet

As Jerry Brunetti would say, "Dump the junk and allow the cavalry to come in." There's much to be learned in this area. Many of the educational materials produced by Soulful Equine can help you with this.

3) Natural trim based on the wild horse

Trim is last on this list because if you apply the other two principles correctly, the trim becomes the least important ingredient, but it is still a big part of the equation.

Other Factors to Consider

Other factors that contribute to soundness in our horses that are important to learn about are:
- ➢ Natural Balance Dentistry®
- ➢ Saddle fit
- ➢ Becoming a balanced, natural rider

SUMMARY OF WHAT TO CONSIDER IF YOU'RE COMING FROM A TRADITIONAL BACKGROUND

1) It's not *only* about the trim. This is an important concept to grasp.
2) It's more about reading the hoof and the situation than it is about the trim.
3) It's a whole horse approach - hoof problems are usually a symptom of an underlying cause.
4) Educate yourself about natural hoof care approaches and keep in mind there are varying opinions.
5) Natural hoof care works because you decide to become more informed and to take action. If you're not up for this respons-ibility, then switching over to natural hoof care may not be for you.
6) Be a strong advocate for barefoot, meaning you're someone who doesn't place metal shoes on a horse. Rather, you under-stand that horses will at times need hoof protection that doesn't prevent the hoof from properly flexing and does not obstruct circulation.
7) You must genuinely care about setting the horse up to allow healing to take place.

I realize this is a lot of information to wrap your head around; however, I wish I had stumbled upon something like this when I got started in natural hoof care many years ago. During that time, the quality of the organizations and the knowledge base was still evolving. It's come a long way since then, and these tips are a great starting point.

Something to consider is that there are many opinions and techniques being applied when it comes to natural hoof care. Do your best to become familiar with the various barefoot trims.

I believe in standing for something even if that means you approach your hoof care using a combination of methods that you've found works - that's what I do.

It's important to understand that each horse and situation is different and blindly applying someone's "standard" approach to a natural trim is not only less than optimal but could be detrimental.

In order for natural hoof care to be successful, it's important to have a wholistic approach to reading the situation at hand. It's important to learn to read the most subtle of signs as well as to have good intuitive abilities.

A note of encouragement for those who don't believe they're capable of intuition or developing that sixth sense - active listening is key. Listen actively to your horse. I probably can't say it enough that "the horse is our best teacher."

I believe the entire package is important to helping our equine partners THRIVE versus just survive.

Horses are unable to THRIVE using only traditional approaches to horse care.

I hope this will get you off to a great start on your journey in natural hoof care. You may want to see our Online Resources section for more information.

NATURAL HOOF CARE FOR THE HORSE GUARDIAN

In this section I introduce you to a high-level guide to use when choosing a natural hoof care professional. There are varying opinions on this subject and what I share with you is, by no means, an exhaustive guide.

CHOOSING A NATURAL HOOF CARE PROFESSIONAL

Choosing a hoof care professional is an art in itself.

Over the years, some natural trimming practices have developed a bad name, and rightfully so. Once you get to the point of choosing a natural hoof care provider, it's a big decision. You're putting the soundness of your horse in someone else's hands. Sometimes when people get to this point, it's a do or die situation, meaning, their horse is already lame for whatever reason, and they feel natural hoof care is their last option.

One thing I've noticed about people who seek out natural hoof care is that they don't make the decision lightly. Usually, they've already done a lot of research and are at the point of being ready to select a trimmer.

Keep in mind no one knows it all. A good hoof care professional is always learning from the horses in her care. There are no better teachers than the horses themselves.

A Few Things to Consider

When going through the process of selecting a professional to work with, always get a referral from someone you trust. This can be difficult because how do you know who to trust? I hope I can help alleviate some of this uncertainty.

I'm a big believer in going through an interview process. Keep in mind it's important to interview more than one natural hoof care specialist.

These questions may be a good place to start.

Ask such questions as:

1) **How long has she been using natural hoof care methods?** If the person you're asking used to be a traditional farrier, it's important that you make it clear that you're not interested in how long she's been shoeing. You want to know how long she's been using natural hoof care methods.

2) **Why did she decide to switch to natural hoof care?** Ask about her personal story. This, in itself, will tell you a lot about a person.

3) **What barefoot trimming method does she use?** Become familiar with the different methods so you can make an informed decision. Rule out any invasive types of trimming. When in doubt, less is more.

4) **What kind of professional training does she have?** I've witnessed individuals falsely claiming to have studied under someone well-known. Often, these people had acquired no education on natural hoof care nor mentored with other natural hoof care professionals. Be sure to ask for references from some of that person's existing clients.

5) **Does she keep up with the latest developments in natural hoof care, and if so, how?** The best way I can describe this is that it's an evolution. We're constantly learning more about how to maintain healthy barefoot horses - from the backyard companion to the professional athlete. There are also strategic methods being applied that can help some of the more severe lameness cases such as navicular, founder and laminitis.

6) **Does she shoe *and* use natural hoof care methods?** If that person says she still shoes (metal shoes), say, "Thank you for your time" and then move on to your next interview.

7) **Does she use a whole-horse approach?** Since most issues don't originate in the hoof, it's important to have this understanding in order to evaluate a situation and recommend the appropriate professional. For example, saddle fit, bodywork, dentist, etc.

8) **Does she have good horsemanship skills?** This one may not be as important to some as it is to me, but what kind of horsemanship skills does she have? It's important that you have someone who treats your horse in a kind manner and with respect.

Keep in mind there may be times that you've hired a hoof care professional and it wasn't a good fit for you and your horse. Don't be afraid to seek out another professional, because it's always important to put your horse first.

All I ask is that you do it in a respectful manner.

IS THERE A NATURAL HOOF CARE PROFESSIONALS LIST?

There are several hoof care organizations and lists available. I would first start with a good recommendation from someone you know. Not only should you know them but know how sound their horses are.

Some natural hoof care organizations rush individuals through a program and favor those who used to be farriers. Just because someone is part of an organization doesn't necessarily mean they're better than someone who isn't. Some of the most well-known, self-taught individuals are successful and well-respected.

Individuals who are the founders of organizations may be self-taught, highly skilled and continuous learners. It's critical not to discount that detail.

This goes back to the importance of references. As of the writing of this book, I've been trimming naturally for nearly ten years.

I was a member of a well-known organization in which so much change occurred over the years that I felt it was affecting the quality of the program. Needless to say, I decided to leave, as did most of their top instructors and trimmers. So over those years, I spent thousands of dollars on an education with an organization that was pretty much dismantled in 2009.

So what happened to all those great hoof care providers? Some branched off and formed their own organizations, some continued trimming without being associated with a particular group and others joined one of the new organizations.

It's been difficult, both as a natural hoof care professional and as a horse guardian, to find a qualified organization to depend on.

Since there are many conflicting views on approaches to natural hoof care, it's caused some unsettled feelings with hoof care professionals and horse guardians. As far as I'm concerned, it's difficult to know where to turn and who to trust.

Some people in the horse industry, or in any industry for that matter, become obsessed with possessing a piece of paper to prove their worth. In other words, they feel they need to be part of an organization, and if that's what works for them, then that's fine. This is a common, socially accepted belief.

> *By no means am I discouraging that; however, most people become easily swayed by, and bound to, a particular trimming organization which can result in closed-mindedness due to the interpretation and teachings of those who control the organization.*

It's important to keep this in mind when selecting a professional. It's not always about the piece of paper.

I know of many horse guardians who hired certified professional farriers who caused their horses to go lame. Some horses became so lame, it resulted in multiple vet bills. It happens, so don't take the task of selecting a professional lightly.

As of this writing, a group I feel comfortable recommending when seeking out a professional is:

American Hoof Association (AHA) – There's a trimmers list on this site. If there isn't a trimmer listed in your area, contact the AHA and ask if they know of any qualified individuals they could recommend who trim near where you live. There are often many trimmers who aren't on a list who are qualified.

> *"Every horse deserves great hoof care and optimal health."*
> ~ Stephanie Krahl

THE IMPORTANCE OF DOING YOUR PART

As a horse guardian, educating yourself is a big part of natural hoof care. An important fact to understand is a natural hoof care professional can only do so much. They can help most horses, but they're limited by the guardians and what they're willing to do to address the underlying issues.

If the guardian isn't willing to address the concerns that the hoof care professional points out (i.e. diet, environment, movement, etc.), then the relationship may be dissolved quickly. It's important that the horse guardian do her part, otherwise, she may not be able to find a natural hoof care professional willing to work with her.

EDUCATE YOURSELF

There are many fantastic resources available that you can use to educate yourself. See the Online Resources section of this book for more information.

NATURAL HOOF CARE - TRIMMING YOUR OWN HORSE

"We are what we repeatedly do. Excellence then, is not an act, but a habit." ~ Will Durant

LEARNING TO TRIM YOUR OWN HORSE – IS IT RIGHT FOR YOU?

Have you ever experienced waking up in the middle of the night thinking about your horse's soundness. You may ask yourself, "Am I doing the right thing? Is there a better way?"

You think about all you've learned from reading information on natural hoof care and watching some great videos. You may have even attended a natural hoof care clinic.

Over the months of searching for a natural hoof care professional you finally find someone who can help you, however, they live too far away to come to your home for regular trims. The frustration builds and then you think, "If only I knew how to trim my own horse."

With the shortage of competent hoof care providers, this is a common thought that enters the mind of many horse guardians. You may have either read or heard that you can easily learn to trim your own horse. Some people think it's as simple as putting a mustang roll on their horses' hooves and that's it. This is a *stereotypical belief*, not only by horse guardians, but also by traditional farriers who usually have limited or no knowledge about natural hoof care.

Depending on how you approach learning to trim, it can produce either positive or negative consequences. It's important to consider all the factors and, of course, your situation before making the leap.

FACTORS TO CONSIDER

Although the idea of trimming your own horse sounds wonderful, there are some factors that may cause you to reconsider.

Will it save you money?

I believe that over the long haul it will save you a lot of money, not to mention the peace of mind it brings. However, the upfront investment can be substantial. For example, it can easily take a dedicated student up to a year to become confident and somewhat competent if you're only trimming your own horse once every 4-5 weeks.

Quality tools will cost $300 or more. If you're taking lessons from a competent hoof care professional - which I highly recommend - you'll need to factor in that cost. Other additional costs would include educational videos, courses and consultation fees.

You have to be physically fit to trim a horse.

You must be in good physical shape if you want to trim your own horse, and it's a different type of physical fitness. For example, I use to play college basketball. Being in top physical condition for playing basketball requires a different type of physical fitness than long distance running. You're using different muscles. One is long distance versus short starts and stops with bursts of energy and strength.

This is similar to trimming horses. You'll be using muscles you probably don't often use. So, even if you *think* you're in great shape, getting under a horse and performing a trim may cause you to think twice.

Trimming a horse's hooves can be dangerous.

Trimming is one of the most dangerous jobs a person can perform when it comes to horses. You're putting yourself and the horse into a vulnerable position. If you don't have great horsemanship skills, it's easy to get into a situation where the horse won't stand for you and you could get injured, even with your gentle backyard pony. People without proper horsemanship skills often become frustrated in this situation, which can lead to injury.

It takes practice to become good.

It can be difficult to build and maintain your skills since your horse only needs to be trimmed once every 4-5 weeks. It takes practice to become good at anything. If you only trim your horse once a month, it can take longer to become skilled and to feel comfortable doing it. Remember you need continuous education, practical application and patience, because it could take a while to become competent.

The most difficult part is learning to read the hoof.

Learning to read the hoof, its shape, wear patterns, etc. is the most difficult part of the trim for anyone to learn. Usually this comes with time and experience. Even competent trimmers still strive to improve this skill. If you're not good at reading what each individual hoof needs, then it's easy to make mistakes that could cause imbalances over time or cause your horse to become sore (either foot or body sore).

There's no cookie cutter approach.

There's no way to teach trimming with the "if this happens then do that" approach. Despite popular belief and what some so-called experts in natural hoof care teach, it's not a cookie cutter approach. Natural hoof care looks at the whole horse. No two horses are the same, and no two hooves are the same.

"There's a big difference between technique and technician." ~ Pat Parelli

YOU'LL KNOW YOU'RE READY WHEN...

It takes a certain type of individual to commit to trimming her own horse. I'm not going to sugar coat it, because I've seen too many people who won't admit to their own limitations. On the other hand, I don't want to discourage you from wanting to learn.

"Confidence is knowing you are prepared." ~Ray Hunt

Here are a few characteristics I usually look for in a potential student:

> **She has dedication** – she must be willing to immerse herself in learning *away from her horse* and separate from her lessons.

> **She wants to be a great student** – *a few characteristics* of a great student are dedication, paying attention, not making assumptions, asking questions, focus and willingness to stay in physical shape between trims and lessons.

> **She understands it's not just about the trim** – the actual trim is a small piece of the puzzle, but an *important* piece. Knowing a technique or two will only get you so far (if you're lucky).

> **She understands that it won't be easy** – frustration and impatience will usually get the best of you if you don't understand that it takes *time and commitment* when learning to trim your own horse.

If you're still interested, the next section covers in detail my recommendations for getting started.

LEARNING TO TRIM YOUR OWN HOI MAKING THE LEAP

In the section of this book on learning to trim your own horse, I covered in detail practical guidelines to consider before fully making a commitment to such an endeavor. For those diehards who would like to make the leap and learn how to trim using the wild horse as their model, you're in the right place. However, if you haven't read the section of this book on learning to trim your own horse, then I would highly recommend you read it first.

SOME PERSONAL STRUGGLES

When I first started researching natural hoof care, I felt like I was somewhat in the dark and didn't know where to turn. I was determined to help my horse, Dillon, become sound again. He was in his mid-teens at the time and had been in shoes almost all of his life.

Back then, the barefoot movement was not as strong as it is today, and yet, even with the wealth of information available, the multitude of horses who've been rehabilitated, and the enhancement of performance horses by going barefoot, many skeptics still exist.

I hope I can help you make the leap a little easier so you can have success in half the time it took me.

HOW I GOT STARTED USING NATURAL HOOF CARE

Many years ago, I was much like you. I knew I needed to do something different. When I think back, I remember I felt like there was something pushing and guiding me to find the answers.

Out of all the information I stumbled upon, I found Jaime Jackson's book *Horse Owners Guide to Natural Hoof Care* (HOG) . As I look down at my copy of the *HOG* sitting on my desk, I feel gratitude because it's the source of information that got me started. It shows its age with its beaten up cover from my carrying it out to the barn in those early years and all the sticky notes protruding out of it.

I also purchased Jaime's book called *The Natural Horse*, which contains his research on wild horses. I feel everyone should consider reading it or at least using it as a reference.

The HOG is what got me started with natural hoof care, along with all the educational bulletins Jaime Jackson published on his website. I devoured every bit of information I could get my hands on. I was determined and committed to help my horse.

My desire, passion and love for learning caused me to make a change and take action.

In the fall of 2003, Pete Ramey's book *Making Natural Hoof Care Work for You* was published. It was an excellent complement to the HOG, and helped fill in a lot of gaps in understanding natural hoof care.

I consider Jaime the founding father of Natural Hoof Care. To this day, I'm thankful that he didn't give up his beliefs despite the backlash he received in the early days before the term "natural hoof care" was in our vocabulary.

From there it's all history and I am where I am today because of my burning desire not to give up, not to allow frustration to get the best of me and to commit to improving my skills and obtaining more knowledge.

DESPITE ALL THE CHALLENGES, YOU STILL WANT TO LEARN – WHERE DO YOU START?

If you got this far reading in this book, you're probably one of the few dedicated individuals cut out for learning to trim your own horse. Below are my recommendations on getting started.

The order is important depending on your situation.

1. Read all my articles on the Soulful Equine website related to natural horse care. Many of the articles have been enhanced and included in this book, but it will be beneficial to keep up on the website articles, clinics and courses we offer.

2. Sign up for the Soulful Equine newsletter and become a member of our community on Facebook so we can keep you

up to date on our latest articles and future e(
grams.

3. Purchase Pete Ramey's DVD set *Under the H(*
serious about learning how to trim using a wild   ...model,
it's important that you actually own this DVD set, not just rent
it. You'll need to refer back to it time and time again. <u>Note:</u>
As of this writing, this DVD set has met the requirements for
20 hours CE credit available for veterinarians and vet techs.

4. Find a competent natural hoof care provider who can first,
get your horse to a maintainable state, and then teach you
how to trim. The *maintainable state* is important.

5. Watch Pete Ramey's *Tools of the Trade* DVD set. I personally
own this, but I believe owning it is optional. See the Online
Resources section for a review I did on this DVD set and my
suggestions on finding a place to rent it.

6. Purchase and read the books and DVDs on natural hoof care
that I recommend in the Online Resources.

7. Once you have completed Pete Ramey's *Under The Horse* DVD
series I would recommend reading through all of the articles
on his website. Some of these articles may be too advanced
for a beginner, so you might want to start with the basics first
as I've recommended. Since he has written his book, many
advances have been made in the natural hoof care movement,
so please keep that in mind and read all the updates for the
book he has provided on his website.

8. This last one is an advanced task, but necessary once you've
followed all the other steps above. Watch the *That's My Horse*
series of DVDs by Pete Ramey. I would recommend renting
them. This series of DVDs contains a wealth of information
when it comes to learning how to better read a horse's hoof,
the situation and knowing what actions to take.

Although this section is packed full of information, I hope it helps
guide you in your natural hoof care journey. The information I
provided is by no means a comprehensive list of the ins and outs of
learning to trim your own horse, so please use this as a starting point
and go from here.

THE NATURAL HOOF CARE SPECIALIST OF THE FUTURE

If we approach our horse care naturally and set up an environment that closely mimics horses in their natural state, hoof care practitioners will be required to be excellent at reading horses' hooves.

When horses move like they would in the wild, they will form hooves that are like no other in domestication. I've noticed this with my own horses since I've had them on a natural boarding track system.

I have to trim my personal horses differently than I trim my customers' horses.

> *My horses' hooves wear beautifully and they forge a hoof through movement that causes me to be mindful of how little I have to do.*

I'm strategic when I apply my tools to one of their hooves.

Rather than look for what to remove, I look for what to leave that they're already maintaining themselves. This is what your ultimate goal should be: a horse that almost maintains their own hooves.

By no means am I advocating that just because you *think* your horse gets enough movement that they don't need hoof care. That's far from the truth.

> *As long as horses are domesticated they will need competent hoof care.*

It's a matter of how often, how much or how little is needed.

This goes back to a golden principle; it's important to know how to read the situation and have the experience, knowledge and ability to know *what* to do, or what *not* to do, depending on the situation.

NATURAL HOOF CARE FOR THE LAMINITIC OR FOUNDERED HORSE

"Anything forced and misunderstood can never be beautiful." Xenophon (430-355 B.C.), Greek general, statesman, philosopher and horseman

The previous chapters of this book covered several starting points when it comes to natural hoof care. This section will provide a different perspective: The horse guardian who has encountered a situation where her horse became laminitic or has foundered.

From a *traditional* point of view, this is usually a difficult subject to address. However, if you're entrenched in natural hoof care, you're aware that these types of cases can be, and are being, rehabilitated almost on a daily basis. It's a controversial subject as far as the root cause of the problem and why it's such an epidemic. In short, my view is that it's man-made.

Since I love to use stories for teaching, I'd like to take this opportunity to share one story that especially touched my life when it comes to foundered horses.

THE SPECIAL PONY WHO STARTED IT ALL

I grew up on a dairy farm in North Central Texas. Like most kids, especially those who live on a farm, I dreamed of having my very own pony. I was about two years old when Thunder came into our family. She was a Shetland pony, palomino in color. Originally, my parents bought her for my sister, who is four years older than me. As time passed and I grew older, the horse bug in me became stronger.

My mom still tells the story about me walking out to Thunder's pen. Thunder would either run over me or bite me and I would still go back for more. How crazy is that? I sometimes wonder about my parents. Why did they let me go out there in the first place? Being farmers, it was probably no big deal to them. I was one of the young-est of seven kids, and since the other six had survived up until then, why worry?

Since my sister never took an interest in the little Palomino, Thunder became my first equine companion. It was like a love/hate relationship between the two of us. Thunder and I had many won-derful times together. She's the first horse who taught me about horse behavior, even at such a young age.

I asked my mother if she remembered how old Thunder was when she passed. We estimated that I was about 12 years old and Thunder was a young 16 years of age.

It's strange, but back then, and even at such a young age, I was somewhat aware that turning horses out on lush green spring grass could cause founder. We probably were not aware at the time that ponies were more susceptible to founder than regular sized horses. Thunder was not exempt and, as in most cases where people lack knowledge, we didn't realize we were the ones causing the problem. Thunder battled with founder for quite some time.

My family was not poor but we also could not spend the money it took to have Thunder trimmed as regularly as she needed. Another thing we probably didn't realize is that she needed to be trimmed more often. Plus, we were not addressing her diet.

When I was 12 years old, my father called the vet to have Thunder put to sleep. I remember the day Thunder passed. We usually kept her in a pen back behind what we called "the big barn" north of our house. My father would not allow me to watch, but I still remember knowing what was going on and standing there watching the vet and my dad walk to the back of the barn where Thunder lived most of her life.

To this day I feel bad that I wasn't by her side when she passed. However, I now know that I can make up for it by doing what I can to help other horses who may be in a similar situation.

More times than not, there is hope. However, in those circum-stances like Thunder's, natural hoof care is often looked upon as some sort of voodoo by traditionalists. All I can say to that is,

> *"Mother Nature and her healing capabilities should never be discounted nor taken lightly." ~ Stephanie Krahl*

HOW DO YOU DO THE VOODOO THAT YOU DO?

Has anyone ever said to you "that's just voodoo" or "it's black magic"? Usually when someone says something like this they're either **1)** ignorant when it comes to the subject at hand or **2)** feeling intimid-ated so they do everything they can to discount the knowledge you have about the subject.

NATURAL HOOF CARE VOODOO

There are countless stories about laminitic or foundered horses where it was suggested by their veterinarian that they be euthanized. Usually the horses that aren't put to sleep survive because their guardians think of them as part of the family. Therefore, out of des-peration, they decide to give natural hoof care a try.

The other stories are usually situations where the horse is thought of as a disposable object, and we all know how that ends.

So, is natural hoof care voodoo? Some traditionally minded indi-viduals including, but not limited to, veterinarians and farriers *still* think so, but in reality this is far from the truth. The mind shift is not where it needs to be in the horse industry, but at least we've seen a lot of change over the last 10 years.

The key to success is implementing basic natural horse care prin-ciples and becoming informed about what it takes to rehabilitate and maintain a laminitic or founder-prone horse.

THEY SHOULD KNOW WHAT THEY'RE DOING, RIGHT?

The common protocol used by most veterinarians for treating lamin-itis is elevating the horse's heels, almost as much as two inches from the ground. This elevation is added on top of heels that may *already* be too high to begin with.

Another common recommendation is to limit movement to a stall, and the diet is usually not properly addressed. This approach does not set up the situation for successfully rehabilitating a laminitic horse.

> *"Just for your information, when someone recommends elevating the heels on your horse, run as fast as you can in the opposite direction! Be sure to take your horse with you." ~Stephanie Krahl*

Due to the wealth of information and effective advancements in the field of laminitis, the practice of elevating the heels is an option that should rarely be considered. Some expert natural hoof care pro-fessionals believe that elevating the heels on laminitic horses is a rare occurrence today, but in many areas of the country it's still a com-mon practice.

I live in one of the largest horse areas in the country, but the knowledge of the professionals is limited. Many are closed-minded to options that have been proven to rehabilitate laminitic horses. So, it's to your advantage to become well informed *especially* for your horse's sake and for the sake of your pocket book.

LOOK AT THE WHOLE PICTURE

Sometimes it's difficult to know who to believe. Many horse guardi-ans listen to other horse guardians who have even less knowledge than they do.

It's important to educate yourself and to listen to your horse. Sometimes it's a matter of needing a little guidance.

If you become part of a mind shift that refuses to treat only symptoms, and instead become an advocate for looking at the whole horse, you'll become part of the solution instead of part of the problem.

Through understanding how to prevent such problems, as well as learning how to address the root cause of issues (instead of only addressing symptoms), the practice of euthanizing horses for laminit-is can become non-existent.

NATURAL HOOF CARE – READING THE SITUATION

"The intuitive mind is a sacred gift and the rational mind is a faithful servant. We have created a society that honors the servant but has forgotten the gift."
~ Albert Einstein

I love the saying "our eyes are the windows to our souls." Let's take that a step further and say, "Our horses' hooves are the windows to their bodies." In the section of this book that covered getting started with natural hoof care, I discussed the importance of looking at the horse from a whole-body standpoint. I mentioned that the hoof is a by-product of almost everything else that's going on in the body.

It's important not to ignore the hoof; instead, use it as a guide to uncover the root cause of issues and become more familiar with what a healthy hoof looks like. Despite the mounds of information now available on identifying a healthy hoof, I still find that this topic is somewhat foreign to the majority of people involved with horses.

A horse's hooves suffer the most when we don't treat their bodies well. The body is extremely intelligent when prioritizing the allocation of nutrients (the same holds true for the human body). The skin, hair and hooves are usually the last to get nutrients, so hoof problems could be an indicator of a problem somewhere else in the body. Thus, the saying,

Our horses' hooves are the windows to their bodies.

An unnatural and inappropriate diet can materialize as deformed or damaged hooves. In fact, the last six months or longer of a horse's general health can often be seen in the hooves.

Many people believe their horse's diet is not poor despite the fact that they're feeding their horses processed feeds, processed supplements and a high sugar and high starch diet. The majority of horses' hooves you're likely to see are *not* healthy. Common deformities have become the norm in the horse industry.

Although natural hoof care has gained popularity for over 10 years, there's still a long way to go when it comes to educating the everyday horse guardian, as well as traditional farriers, about strategies for identifying a healthy hoof and how to maintain it.

HEALTHY HOOVES SHARE SIMILAR CHARACTERISTICS

Horses' hooves can grow in a variety of shapes based on individual conditions, genetics, etc., but healthy hooves share similar characteristics.

Healthy hooves are smooth with no rings or distortions in the hoof wall.

If you see ridges or rings (also referred to as *event rings*) of any kind on the outside of the hoof wall, it's important that you identify the cause. The humorous part of that statement is that rings in the hoof wall have become something that most horse guardians and traditional farriers don't pay attention to.

The important thing for you to know right now is that you must pay attention to it and *one* of the biggest causes is an unnatural and inappropriate diet for that particular horse. Rings in the hoof wall can provide a wealth of information not only related to diet, stress, etc. but also hoof dysfunction.

The hooves should not easily chip and the hoof wall/horn should not easily break off.

I'm referring to barefoot horses that are kept on a competent natural hoof care program. There are some exceptions to this rule, but once you transition your horse to barefoot and you've addressed the three key areas, which include, **movement**, **diet** *and a* **proper barefoot trim**, then this statement should hold true.

If you continue to have problems with your horse going barefoot, or the characteristics of a healthy hoof are still not obvious to you in your own horse, then you're missing one of those key ingredients.

It's important to educate yourself. The barefoot movement is continuing to evolve and we're learning new things every day on what works and what doesn't work for the *domesticated* horse.

Hooves should have short toes & low heels.

A *healthy* horse is not meant to have hooves that look like duck feet. I use this analogy because I see many shod horses, as well as tradition- ally trimmed barefoot horses, that have long or under run heels and a flared long toe. Also, horses are not meant to walk around like they're in ladies high-heeled shoes.

If you would like more information on measurements of wild horse hooves I would highly recommend Jaime Jackson's book *The Natural Horse* where he provides information on hoof shape and form in detail. It's an exceptional book if you're looking for measurement information.

Granted, the measurements in that book were taken on wild horses, but always remember that our "model" and "guide" is the wild horse. Keep in mind, there's not just one wild horse model. Hoof form can vary depending on the horse's terrain and environment.

Your horse should have a nice "heel first" landing in order to continue to stay sound.

It's your natural hoof care professional's job to guide the hoof and set it up properly for a heel first landing. I highly recommend that you learn how to spot what this looks like since the norm in the horse industry is usually a toe first landing.

Ask a competent hoof care professional to help you learn to have an eye for how your horse is landing. This is important: I can't stress it enough. If they're landing toe first, there are multiple reasons for it and one can be linked to diet.

Another is linked to improper development of the back of the foot, which is common in domesticated horses. Thrush is often a cause that's overlooked as well.

If a horse is landing toe first, this is a sign of lameness. A horse *is* in pain, for whatever reason, if their landing this way. They also have to compensate and exert more energy in order to land comfortably.

Healthy hooves should not have flaring or a stretched white line.

A stretched white line can be an indicator of an unnatural and inappropriate diet, imbalanced hooves, etc. This goes back not only to diet but also properly guiding the hoof so that over time the horse develops a healthy toe length and an overall balanced hoof.

A nice straight angle of growth is important in a healthy hoof. It's best to follow the new angle from the upper 2 inches of growth from the coronary band. This is important in order to keep flares under control, but it can be detrimental if someone becomes "flare happy" by trying to remove all the flare from a hoof in one trim. That approach can cause thinning of the hoof wall and weakening of the overall hoof structure.

A competent natural hoof care professional will know how to safely address flares as well as help you identify the root cause. I can't stress this enough. If your horse continues to flare between trims, it's important to figure out the underlying cause.

Again, an unnatural and inappropriate diet is usually the culprit if the horse is getting proper routine maintenance trims. It could also be caused by improper trimming methods or by your horse's confirmation.

There are no hard and fast rules with flare. Sometimes flaring is justified. Again, I want to stress that a competent natural hoof care professional will know how to properly read the hoof.

Cindy "Hawk" Sullivan wrote an article that would be worth your time to read called *Going Nuts Over Flares?* You can find a reference to her website in our Online Resources section.

The frog should be large and calloused.

The "large" part of that statement about the frog is true; however frogs will vary in consistency based on terrain. In dry terrain, they will have a leather look to them and will be wider and flatter. In wet weather, the frog will have a more rubbery look to it and will also be fuller versus flat.

Most unhealthy hooves have a narrow frog along with contracted heels. When you see a horse with a skinny, underdeveloped frog and contracted heels, this is a sure sign that the horse is not landing properly and getting enough stimulation to the back of the foot. This means the horse is landing toe first.

These are just a few tips for the horse guardian. Although it's not an exhaustive list, these are some key attributes to look for in spotting a healthy hoof.

PART VI: THE POWER OF REFLECTION

Sometimes the hardest thing for us humans to do is look at ourselves before we blame others for our situation or circumstances. That's much easier than reflecting inward on those elements of ourselves that horses are masters at feeling and reading. Horses truly are our mirrors.

Throughout the remaining chapters of this book, I will share with you how your relationship with horses has a lot to do with self-improvement and self-discovery. So sit back and enjoy some of the following concepts that might help improve your relationship with your horse.

HORSEMANSHIP AND LEADERSHIP

"Horsemanship can be obtained naturally through psychology, communication, and understanding, versus mechanics, fear and intimidation." ~ Pat Parelli

HOW TO OVERCOME YOUR THREE GREATEST HORSEMANSHIP CHALLENGES

Where are the holes that are getting in the way of you obtaining excellence with horses? Becoming excellent in anything takes dedication and time. Master horsemen will take more time putting "foundation before specialization," and they understand the importance of the little things.

Just imagine you're at a horsemanship 101 clinic. It's the first day of the clinic and the clinician tells everyone to *saddle up* and join him in the arena in 30 minutes. You already have your horse in hand so you lead her over to your trailer and begin politely saddling her.

As you're saddling your horse you notice two trailers down from you a young woman attempting to saddle her horse. The first thing you notice is that the horse is tied long. As you try to get over the fact that the horse is tied long, you also notice the incorrectly tied knot and that the rope halter is about to slip over her nose.

As the horse is moving around, the person tries to throw the saddle up onto the horse's back.

*The horse is so offended by the rudeness of her human that
she pins her ears and attempts to bite.*

The person hits the horse on the face and continues saddling.

On it goes with the person grabbing the back cinch and buckling it up before putting on the front cinch. The horse voices her opinion about the situation by dancing around. By some act of God the person finally gets the front cinch snug enough on the horse to head over to the arena.

She enters the arena where about 10 other individuals are riding around and the clinician is waiting to call the class into session. You ride in behind her as she leads her horse into the arena.

Everyone is riding around as she attempts to mount her horse. The horse continues to dance around and as she's trying to get on, her saddle slips onto the side of her horse. She keeps trying to mount up and then the clinician yells to her, "Get that horse out of here and properly cinch her up! If that saddle slipped under her belly you could kill us all in here!!!"

This is not a joke – I've witnessed similar crazy events. What's wrong with the situation I described to you? I'd be willing to bet that you can point out many problems with this scenario.

HERE'S THE GOOD NEWS

There is hope. I have to continue to remind myself that not everyone chooses to move toward achieving excellence with horses. Most people are happy with just getting by and not getting killed. I've come to realize that not everyone desires to have a high-level relationship with a horse.

Here's something to consider: What if you were working on the path to excellence and, by default, that allowed you to be safer and nearly eliminate ever having a "bad" horse day.

For 10+ years, I've noticed three of the toughest hurdles people face with improving their horsemanship. I've also struggled with these same hurdles, so don't think I was exempt, because I wasn't.

Awareness is the first step to causing change.

So here are some ways to get over what I believe are three of the toughest horsemanship hurdles. The sooner you decide to improve in these areas, the sooner you can have more fun and stay safer with your horse. By no means am I saying it's going to be easy. If it were easy, everyone would do it. But it's also not as hard as it appears right now.

OLD HABITS DIE HARD

I have to admit, I have some poor horsemanship habits that **1)** I may not be aware of and **2)** I'm aware of and I'm working towards changing.

Since I'm a dedicated student of horses, there are times I may catch something I did on one of my videos that I had no idea I was doing. I wasn't conscious of it. This happens to all of us.

Video may be one of the more powerful ways to observe yourself without feeling like a failure or being offended because one of your friends pointed out the fact that you're a blockhead around your horse. Remember, a good friend will be honest with you, and they won't sugar coat it because it could mean the difference between you staying safe or getting hurt.

The best tip I can provide on interrupting old habits, after becoming aware of them, is to be willing to make a change. And the biggest motivating factor to make that change will be your burning desire to have a *great* relationship with your horse and to have good horsemanship habits.

MONKEY SEE MONKEY DO

Think back to the situation I described at the beginning of this sec-tion. What if the person observing the situation was new to horses? She might think that there's nothing wrong with tying a horse long or with the halter about to come over the horse's nose. She may think that it's okay to hit a horse and that what she observed is the proper way to saddle a horse, not realizing that there were many safety con-cerns in that scenario as well as a disconnect in the person's relationship with her horse.

Setting both good and bad examples are extremely powerful, so why not choose to make it a habit to set good examples?

This is just a simple example, but this type of *Monkey See Monkey Do* mentality happens more often than not in the horse industry. The best tip I can think of providing when it comes to this is to be careful where you get your information. Just because you saw someone else do something with a horse, don't blindly accept it; always question "why?" It's also important not to discount it if you have ill feelings about how someone is treating a horse.

When learning something new, observe different ways and then compare techniques. You'll know when the right one resonates with you. When observing how someone treats a horse, don't allow yourself to be swayed just because that person is a trainer or an "expert." Keep in mind that many top trainers have poor horsemanship skills.

There's a big difference between a trainer and a horseman and between training a horse versus developing a horse.

READING HORSES AND HORSE SITUATIONS

I saved *reading horses and the situation* for last because I believe this is the most difficult of the three. Learning to read and understand horse behavior can be a life long endeavor, but it's well worth pursuing. This is the area that separates the *true horseman* from the mediocre trainer, those who use force with horses or someone just wanting to get by.

Learning how to use psychology rather than fear and intimidation, is not normal for most equine enthusiasts, especially if they think it's too hard and it will get in the way of a blue ribbon or winning a futurity.

Mastering the art of putting the horse's noble nature first, and relating to them through their mind *before* asking for the physical, is not for everyone. The best tip I can provide here is to study.

Study those who you know have a special connection with horses.

Observe them, learn from them and most of all learn from your horse.

Learn to listen to your horse more than you listen to humans and you'll find the answers.

Reading horses and situations is the most important area, and it's constantly overlooked. The better someone becomes at it, the safer they will be around horses.

A few other concepts to consider are as follows:

> ➢ A great technique is not always the answer
> ➢ Become a better problem solver

You don't have to be an amazing trainer to be an amazing horseman. But you do have to make a change if you seek excellence with horses. For master horsemen, it may be minor tweaks and for others, like me, we have a long road ahead. I don't know about you, but I'm enjoying every step.

The more you learn and develop yourself, the more your horsemanship skills will improve. Through learning more about you, you'll learn more about your horse. I know, sounds weird, but it works. So get going and pick one of the three things I mentioned and see if there are areas in your horsemanship you can improve.

WHY HORSEMANSHIP SKILLS REQUIRE PERSONAL DEVELOPMENT

I've been a dedicated student of the horse ever since I can remember. Having horses in my life is the very reason that helps me get out of bed each morning. They're a special part of my life and I feel I need them like I need air to breathe.

Over 10 years ago I stumbled upon a concept called natural horsemanship. The more I learned about becoming aware and connected with horses the more I grew as an individual.

Due to my passion for excellence, it's caused a change in me that I didn't see coming.

When I first started studying natural horsemanship, I got into it because I thought I wanted to learn how to become a better trainer, when in reality I started down a path that was unexpected. Little did I know that I would learn to carefully select my words, for example, no longer using the word's "train" and "break" when they relate to horses.

Now, when I hear those words, I have a completely different feeling. When I hear someone say, "That's a broke horse" I just cringe. The word "broke" has a negative connotation and the people who still say it, more than likely, haven't yet found that true connection they *can* have with horses.

Over the years, I've learned the importance of thoughts and words and how powerful they are. I now understand the difference between a partner and a mindless robot. I believe that developing horses is much better than "training" them.

I'm constantly working on my skill at reading horses and situations. This acquired skill has kept me safe and I can't remember the last time I've had a *bad horse day*. It rarely happens.

By honing this skill over the years, I've changed my mind about a lot of things, especially competitions. I can hardly stand to watch what horses have to put up with in some events.

I often have people say to me, "I bet you can't go to a horse event without noticing the horses' hooves and how they land."

That's a true statement, but the first thing I do is read the horse, and then that usually leads to me noticing pain and discomfort somewhere else. It takes me about two seconds from there to read the kind of relationship a horse and horse guardian have with each other.

Horses are excellent judges of character and they usually have us sized up from a mile away. It's in their DNA. I sometimes remind myself that my horses probably used to look at me like a dumb human, but now I do everything I can to have a partnership with them. A partnership is not a one-sided relationship.

On multiple occasions, I've wished that I had the ability to help someone see and feel, just for a few minutes, through their horse's eyes. That alone would cause a change and shift in their actions and feelings toward their horse.

Our horses are a mirror image of us. Anytime you're around a horse or have a horse in hand, they'll reflect back to you the energy you're giving off.

Have you ever seen a horse act differently depending on who's handling her or who's around her? A horse reads and feels our energy. They don't just read our body language like most people believe. Our thoughts can also radiate through our body, so it's a good idea to be mindful of your thoughts when you're around a horse. So why am I going into all this stuff?

One of the biggest keys to you successfully having a naturally healthy horse has to do with the relationship between you and your horse.

As you've probably experienced, a horse can cause you to feel every human emotion imaginable. The way I look at it, the more I cared for myself and grew as an individual, the better I was able to manage all of those emotions.

If you choose to pursue the natural horse route, the journey, independent of your horse, will lead you down a road to self-development and personal fulfillment that will, ultimately, make you the human your horse wants you to be.

THE HORSE, OUR MOST NOBLE FRIEND

"For lack of a better word, I've taken to calling this the horse's spirit. The older I get, the more I have come to believe that this aspect of the horse is the most important and the most overlooked." ~ Tom Dorrance

As I was out walking the horse track, putting out hay and doing the regular poop-scooping regimen, I thought to myself, what am I going to write about during the week of Christmas?

I usually do some of my best brainstorming and come up with most of my ideas while I'm out doing my regular equine chores in the mornings. What immediately popped into my head was this question, "What do you think about around Christmas?" The first thing that came to mind was my father who passed away in 2002.

I continued to ponder how I would write about my father and not cause everyone to cry. I also thought about how I would tie it in with something equine related. A good friend of mine then came to mind.

Around May of 2006, this friend, who used to work for the Dallas Morning News, asked to interview me about my father's death and our relationship. Leslie is her name and she wrote a wonderful article that was published May 22, 2006 called *Passed on – but not gone... A gesture, a scent. It's as if your loved one is right beside you.*

Being the pack rat that I am, I went looking for a copy of the article that Leslie had given me. Sure enough I found it delicately placed along with some other special items of mine. As I read through the article it caused me to think back on some of the nice moments my father and I had during the last two years prior to his passing. Some of my siblings saw my father in a much different light, but they didn't get to know the man I came to know those last two years.

My father was a farmer all his life, and he was wise when it came to farming and animals. He had a love for the land and for animals like most farmers have and I believe he passed that love on to me, for which I will be forever grateful.

However, I have a slightly different love than he did for what I consider the most noble of animals - THE HORSE.

The bond that my horses helped to create between my father and me was something magical. There's something about the horse that's so special that I believe it can cause relationships to mend as well as help us to grow as human beings.

My horses and the love surrounding them gave me the opportunity to grow even closer to my father before he passed. It's interesting how life sets up opportunities for us to learn lessons. In my case, many lessons have come from being around horses.

The horse is a gift each of us should cherish, respect and pay tribute to. I dedicate this story and book to those soulful creatures who have passed before us and, to our most noble friend...

THE HORSE.

GRATITUDE

Often times it takes you losing an important piece of life before real-izing that it's gone forever - that moment in time that can never be replicated or replaced. All my life I've had the drive to move forward, achieve more, learn more, and do better - continuous improvement. It took years of pressuring myself into taking a step back, looking at what I've accomplished, and pausing for a moment of gratitude.

Now, I make sure I take time out of each day and dedicate it to that powerful value I hold close - gratitude. I believe the power of sincere gratitude reaps a multitude of benefits, one being that it helps remind us - day in and day out - that it could be worse and that it's not all that bad. The act of taking time each day for being grateful for one thing, makes us realize we have so much more to be grateful for. The good things somehow start to multiply and then we have difficulty choosing which thing to be grateful for that day.

No one gets to where they are in life without help along the way. Sometimes it's a stranger who comes into your life for a brief period - often times showing up at the perfect moment when you needed someone most. Then there are those with whom you become friends, but not for the long haul. They come into your life for a specific pur-pose unknown to you or them. Sometimes you don't know their impact until years later. And then there are the ones who are in it for the long haul - the ones who stand the test of time. They're with you through thick and thin. These people are usually few and far between, and the value and quality they provide to your life is price-less - few offer this enormous benefit.

There are many people who have directly and indirectly had an impact on my life - some still do. Without them putting their imprint on me, it would have been different, so much so, in fact, that this book, as well as Soulful Equine, may never have been created.

As I take a look back at my life, the first person who helped me start my journey with horses was my father - Martin Krahl. As you read in the last part of the book, he has since passed. In November 2012, it will have been 10 years. That sounds like a long time, but it goes by in the blink of an eye.

My father was always supportive of my love and passion for horses. He and I were so much alike. He had a love for animals, farming, and a work ethic that allowed him to get through some of the toughest times of raising 7 kids on a farmer's budget. Although, like most relationships, we had our ups and downs, I owe much of my gratitude to my father. Without his support for my passion for horses, I believe I wouldn't be as happy as I am today, nor would I be sharing the wealth of knowledge with you that I've acquired over a lifetime of study. I'm grateful that my father taught me the meaning of having a strong work ethic. He was by no means perfect, far from it in fact, but he, like you and I, had lessons to learn in life.

Ever since I can remember, I've said, "If you don't have your health, you don't have anything." Over the years I've had many health care practitioners come and go, but one in particular I hold dear to my heart. He not only got me on the road to continuous and optimal health, but he's played a significant role in my overall progress in life for the past 13 years. His name is Dr. Rob Parker with Parker Health Solutions (his website: www.parkerhealthsolutions.com). If there are angels on earth, he comes close. The biggest part in moving forward in life is not only about physical health of the body, but first and foremost about your spiritual and energetic well-being. Rob has helped me remove many obstacles in my path that would have otherwise prevented me from moving forward on my life's journey.

I've always been an admirer of people who are artists. Photography is an art and I would like to thank my sister, Lynn McKay, for all the pictures she takes when she comes to visit - she's a wonderful photographer. Lynn took the photographs included in this book. She has helped get me through some tough times in my life, and she's a wonderful house sitter as well. If Lynn wasn't willing to take her vacations at my home, it would be more difficult to get away and go to clinics, travel, and experience new adventures as they relate to horses. It's hard to find someone you can trust with your animals when you have to be absent from them for periods of time. I can't express enough gratitude for Lynn's support of my love for horses and animals. If you have a sister or brother like Lynn, go give them a hug, or call them right now because they deserve to know how much you appreciate them.

Although I've had many mentors and formal training when it comes to horses, one person in particular I'm grateful for is Bruce Goode. Bruce is a natural hoof care trimmer (his website: www.hooftrack.com), who played an important role in helping me move forward with trimming my own and other people's horses. Bruce allowed me to tag along with him for a few months one summer when he went to trim client's horses. I learned a lot during those few months, not only about how to become a more efficient and effective trimmer, but also about safety and dealing with difficult customers and horses. Had I not accompanied Bruce during those few months, an important chain of events would not have occurred that had a great impact on Soulful Equine materializing.

Many people played a part in helping this book come to life. Those who stepped up and were so kind to give me honest, well edited feedback that brought more clarity to my message are as follows: Mary Tousley, Mo Vear, Kathy Kirsh, Garry Moore, Sreelatha Surendranathan, Sharon Tousley, and Susan Chambers (her website: sdc-sage-editing.com). Susan is a professional editor who, after we all went through the book with a fine-toothed comb, gave me some great feedback with a soft edit of the entire book. Without the collective effort of everyone involved, my writing would not shine nearly as bright in order to have a greater reach.

Each and every horse that's come into my life brought forth a piece of their energy into this book. Without those wonderful teachers, none of this would have been possible. Most of all, I'm grateful for my three personal horses - Faith, Dillon and Ransom. They've taught me so much and there's still so much more to learn.

The most important person I would like to express my deepest gratitude to is Sharon Tousley. Sharon goes above and beyond as a partner in Soulful Equine's success and in my own success. She's my personal peer editor and is my greatest asset as a writer. Had it not been for her support and tolerance of my crazy ambitious character, and passion for horses, Soulful Equine may never have existed. Everyone needs a Sharon in their life.

To my fellow horse lovers and readers of Soulful Equine, thank you for your support. Feel free to contact me in writing at any time at soulfulequine.com

Keep it soulful and always remember to put your horse's noble nature first.

Stephanie Krahl
Texas

ABOUT THE COVER

Have you ever experienced an event in your life where you needed something and it appeared in the nick of time - the stars seemed to align and allowed synchronicity to occur?

That's what happened when I stumbled upon a talented artist in Texas named **Laurie Justus Pace**. I picked up the June, 2011 publication of *Horseback Magazine*, read an article about her, and fell in love with her artwork at first glance.

Since we had a shoe-string budget, it was difficult finding the *perfect* image to reside on our front cover. We knew it needed to be special, but we didn't want it to be like other natural horse care books that had a picture of a wild horse. Although that's beautiful, and it crossed our minds, it didn't feel like the perfect fit.

Even though Laurie's artwork sells at premium prices, she graciously offered to donate an image (of my choice!) for the cover. She has an eye for the spirit of the horse that radiates through her artwork like no other. The image selected is called *Rebirth of Color*.

I would like to encourage you to visit her website at www.ellepace.com and her blog at www.lauriepace.blogspot.com You will not be disappointed. Who knows, you may find that "perfect" piece of art for that special project or person at the perfect time.

Keep it soulful,
Stephanie Krahl
Texas

ONLINE RESOURCES

Due to the large amount of information about keeping a naturally healthy horse, this book had to be considerably condensed. The intent was not to give you step by step instructions, but instead to provide a guide that would instill a solid foundation to jump-start you with natural horse care.

To assist you on learning more about what was discussed in this book, I made a resources area on our website, Soulful Equine. It provides a wealth of information, some of which includes:

> ➢ A list of Soulful Equine articles and reports to enhance your understanding of the concepts discussed in this book.
> ➢ Recommended books, magazines, audios and videos to help further your education on natural horse care.
> ➢ Natural hoof care resources around the web.
> ➢ More on equine dentistry and various other alternative modalities you can look into.
> ➢ Information on putting a non-toxic fly control program in place that works.

The information contained in these online resources is free to those who buy this book. To get access, all you have to do is go to www.soulfulequine.com and send us an email letting us know you purchased the book.

INDEX

ABOUT THE AUTHOR

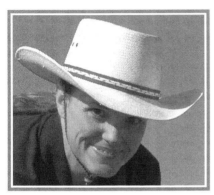 **Stephanie Krahl** developed a passion for horses at a very young age, and they've played a key role in her life ever since. It started at the age of two with a pony named Thunder, and as a kid she read everything she could get her hands on about horses, from caring for them to learning more about horsemanship.

At the age of nine, with the guidance of her father, she started her first horse under saddle and learned the importance of building a strong relationship with a horse.

Her ability to understand and connect with horses has always been an innate quality. It wasn't until later in life that her education and experience in human health and wellness played a huge role in transitioning her horse care mindset from a traditional to a natural approach. Little did she know that, as a teenager, when a family friend taught her the basics of trimming her own horses, it would come into play later on in Stephanie's life.

When it comes to horses, Stephanie refuses to settle for mediocre. That passion for learning, and constantly seeking out the best for the horse, has opened up doors far beyond her imagination.

Her degree in Computer Science and Mathematics set up opportunities to become an above average problem solver. Since everything pertaining to horses requires great problem solving skills, it has played a significant role in analyzing, observing and seeking out the best in natural horse care.

Stephanie is a natural horse care specialist, a writer, teacher, coach, all-around web geek, and CEO and co-founder of Soulful Equine, who teaches horse guardians about natural horse concepts that help their horse THRIVE. She consistently contributes educational articles on natural horse care at www.soulfulequine.com and regularly provides coaching services as a natural horse care specialist. If you want a thriving equine, sign up for Stephanie's newsletter at www.soulfulequine.com.

CONNECT WITH STEPHANIE

www.soulfulequine.com
twitter.com/soulfulequine
facebook.com/soulfulequine

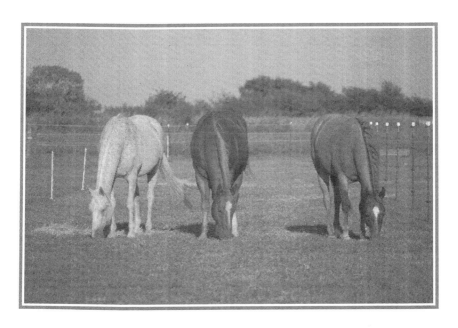

The horses of Soulful Equine from left to right: Faith, Dillon and Ransom

SOULFUL EQUINE™
Helping Your Horse Thrive™
www.soulfulequine.com

Made in the USA
Lexington, KY
04 April 2014